KNOW YOUR MOUTH

THE ESSENTIAL GUIDE TO UNDERSTANDING TEETH ....IN 1 HOUR!!......

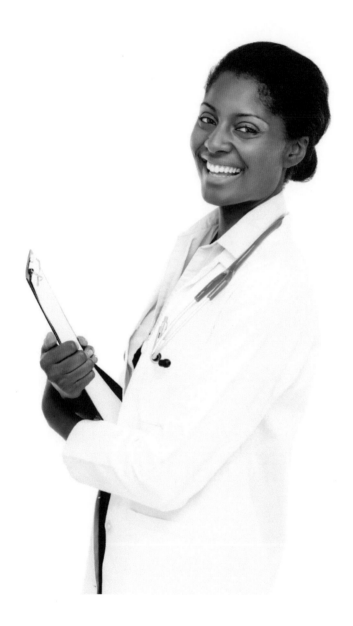

KNOW YOUR MOUTH

THE ESSENTIAL GUIDE TO UNDERSTANDING TEETH ....IN 1 HOUR!!......

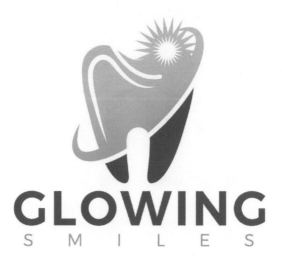

GLOWING
S M I L E S

CONTENTS

...WHO IS DR. LEE?...

DR. JONATHAN SHAUN LEE IS A DENTAL SURGEON WHO GRADUATED FROM **GUY'S AND ST. THOMAS' HOSPITAL** IN 2001.

PRIOR TO BECOMING A DENTIST, HE STUDIED **SPORTS NUTRITION** AT KINGS COLLEGE LONDON FOR 3 YEARS WHILST TAKING A LONG BREAK FROM HIS DENTAL STUDIES.

IN 1998, DR. LEE GRADUATED FROM KINGS COLLEGE LONDON WITH **A BACHELOR OF SCIENCE DEGREE IN SPORTS NUTRITION AND MEDICAL SCIENCE.** HE SPENT A FEW YEARS THEREAFTER WORKING AS A **NUTRITIONIST AND PERSONAL TRAINER.**

IN 2002, HE MOVED FROM HIS HOMETOWN IN LONDON TO THE WEST MIDLANDS WHERE HE STARTED WORKING IN GENERAL PRACTICE AS A DENTAL SURGEON.

DR. LEE HAS **OVER 20 YEARS** EXPERIENCE IN THE FIELD OF DENTISTRY, AND HAS TO DATE TREATED OVER 180,000 PATIENTS.

HE IS A STRONG BELIEVER IN POSTGRADUATE EDUCATION AND IN ADDITION TO HIS MANY YEARS IN PRACTICE, DR. LEE HAS ALSO COMPLETED A NUMBER OF POSTGRADUATE COURSES COVERING A WIDE RANGE OF DENTAL SPECIALITIES.

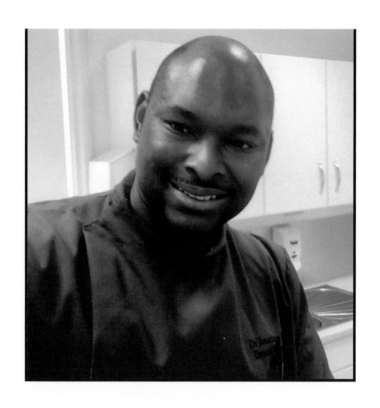

DR JONATHAN S. LEE BDS, BSc

SO WHAT WILL YOU GET FROM THIS BOOK??

"IN A NUTSHELL, THIS BOOK WAS WRITTEN FOR ANYONE WITH A BASIC INTEREST IN TEETH, GUMS, AND DENTAL HEALTH. DR. LEE'S ULTIMATE AIM WAS TO PROVIDE THE READER WITH A GENERAL OVERVIEW OF DENTISTRY WITHOUT COVERING SPECIFIC TOPICS IN TOO MUCH DETAIL.

SO WHAT DOES THAT MEAN???

WELL PUT IT THIS WAY, AFTER TREATING NEARLY 200,000 PATIENTS DURING HIS 20 YEAR CAREER, DR. LEE COULDN'T HELP BUT NOTICE THE MAJORITY OF HIS PATIENTS ASKING THE SAME QUESTIONS TIME AND TIME AGAIN.

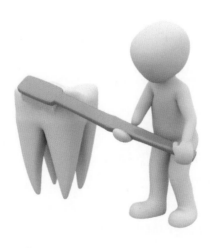

LET'S TAKE A LOOK
AT THESE QUESTIONS

"DOCTOR, WHY DO I NEED A FILLING IF MY TEETH DON'T HURT?"

"DOCTOR, WHY ARE MY GUMS BLEEDING ALL THE TIME?"

"DOCTOR, I'M GETTING TOOTHACHE BUT I DON'T KNOW WHERE THE PAIN IS COMING FROM?"

"DOCTOR, WHY ARE MY TEETH GETTING LOOSE?"

"DOCTOR, HOW LONG ARE FILLINGS SUPPOSED TO LAST? MINE KEEP BREAKING!

"DOCTOR, IS THIS GONNA HURT??"

"DOCTOR, WHY DOES MY BREATH SMELL?"

"DOCTOR, I BRUSH MY TEETH ALL THE TIME. WHY DO I KEEP GETTING HOLES IN THEM?"

"DOCTOR, WHY ARE MY GUMS RECEDING?"

"DOCTOR, WHY DO I GET JAW ACHE EVERY TIME I WAKE UP?"....

"DOCTOR, CAN I GET IMPLANTS ON THE NHS?

"DOCTOR, WHY DO YOU LEAVE THE ROOM EVERY TIME YOU TAKE AN X-RAY?"

"DOCTOR, WHY ARE MY TEETH TURNING YELLOW?"

"DOCTOR, IS IT BETTER TO HAVE THIS DONE PRIVATELY OR ON THE NHS ?"

"DOCTOR, HOW COME MY FRIEND'S DENTURES ARE TIGHT AND COMFORTABLE BUT MINE KEEP FALLING OUT?"

"DOCTOR, I HAD MY TOOTH OUT 2 DAYS AGO BUT I'M STILL IN PAIN. WHAT'S GOING ON??"

"DOCTOR, DO ROOT FILLINGS WORK? MY FRIEND HAD IT ONCE AND ENDED UP LOSING HIS TOOTH!"

"DOCTOR, THESE ANTIBIOTICS DON'T WORK! WHY AM I STILL GETTING TOOTHACHE?"

"DOCTOR, HOW OFTEN SHOULD I VISIT THE DENTIST?"

"DOCTOR, WHY DO MY JAW MUSCLES HURT EVERY MORNING?

"I HATE DENTISTS!! AM I THE ONLY ONE??"

BELIEVE IT OR NOT, THESE ARE QUESTIONS MOST DENTISTS GET ASKED ON A REGULAR BASIS!!

AND MY GUESS IS THAT YOU CAN PROBABLY RELATE TO SOME OF THEM, **ESPECIALLY THE LAST ONE.**

THE GOOD NEWS IS THAT THIS BOOK ANSWERS ALL OF THESE QUESTIONS IN ADDITION TO COVERING EVERYTHING YOU NEED TO KNOW ABOUT TEETH, GUMS, POLITICS, AND MODERN DENTISTRY.

BUT HERE'S THE BEST PART!

IT SHOULDN'T TAKE YOU MORE THAN AN HOUR TO READ FROM BEGINNING TO END.

SO WITHOUT FURTHER ADO, LET'S GET STUCK IN.

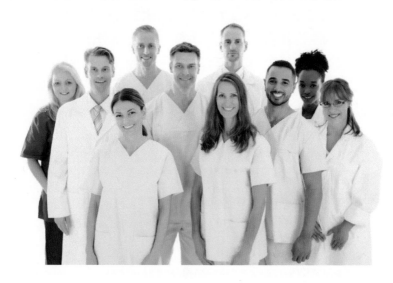

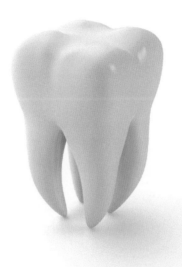

CHAPTER 1

WHAT IS A TOOTH?

SO, WHAT ARE
TEETH...EXACTLY?

- Quite simply, 'teeth' can be defined as a set of hard, bonelike structures rooted in sockets which make up part of the jaw(s).

- Teeth are the hardest substances in the human body. We use our teeth for biting and chewing our food. They also play an important role in speech and appearance.

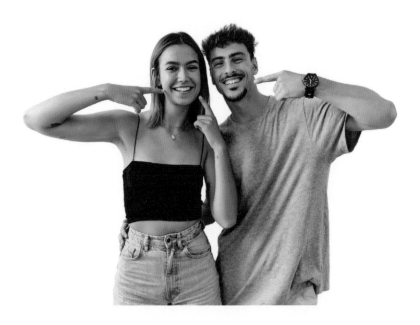

..AND WHAT ARE
TEETH MADE OF?..

ENAMEL	DENTINE
The enamel is the white tissue that covers and protects your teeth. It is the most visible part of a tooth. Nothing in the body is harder than enamel.	*Dentine is the hard, yellow-coloured substance that supports the enamel and protects the pulp.*
PULP	**CEMENTUM**
The innermost region of a tooth consists of a pulp. The pulp is a jelly-like substance which contains nerves and blood vessels.	*This is the hard layer that coats and protects the root of your tooth lying underneath your gums.*

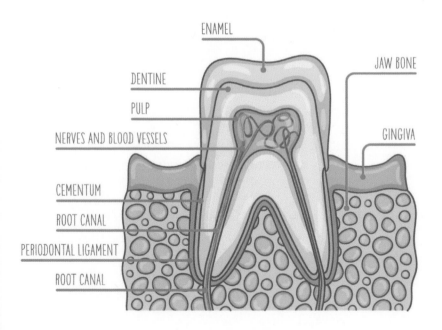

THERE ARE FOUR
TYPES OF TEETH

INCISORS (8 in Total)	**CANINES** (4 in Total)
The incisor teeth are at the front of the mouth and classically have a flat edge designed for shearing, biting and cutting.	The canines (or eye-teeth) are the longest teeth, located next to the incisors. They are the most stable teeth and are designed for tearing food.
PREMOLARS (8 in Total)	**MOLARS** (8-to-12 in Total)
These teeth are located between the canines and the molars. Their function is to both tear and chew food. Kids don't have premolar teeth.	Molar teeth are at the back of the mouth and are designed to chew food. Most of us have 8 molars, but a 3rd set of molars erupt in most adults between 18-20 and over.

TYPES OF TEETH

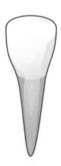 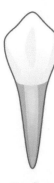 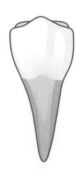 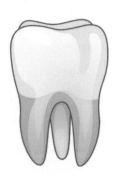

Incisor Canine Premolar Molar

HOW MANY TEETH
DO WE HAVE?

- Throughout life, we have 2 sets of teeth. Our first set consists of 20 teeth and are commonly referred to as **'milk teeth'** or 'baby teeth.' They start to appear in our mouths from the age of **6 months old**. The last milk tooth erupts at around 24 months. Therefore, by the time a child is **2 years old**, he/she would likely have a full set of milk teeth.

- **From the age of 6 years old**, these milk teeth start to become loose and drop out. Over time, they are gradually replaced with bigger teeth which remain in our jaws for the rest of our lives. This second set of teeth are our 'permanent' or **'adult' teeth**. In total, there are **32 adult teeth**.

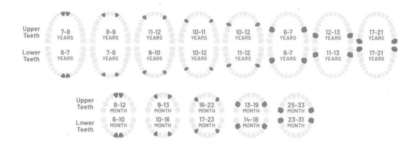

WHEN DO OUR TEETH MAKE AN APPEARANCE?

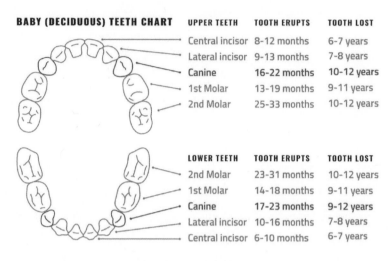

BABY (DECIDUOUS) TEETH CHART

UPPER TEETH	TOOTH ERUPTS	TOOTH LOST
Central incisor	8-12 months	6-7 years
Lateral incisor	9-13 months	7-8 years
Canine	16-22 months	10-12 years
1st Molar	13-19 months	9-11 years
2nd Molar	25-33 months	10-12 years

LOWER TEETH	TOOTH ERUPTS	TOOTH LOST
2nd Molar	23-31 months	10-12 years
1st Molar	14-18 months	9-11 years
Canine	17-23 months	9-12 years
Lateral incisor	10-16 months	7-8 years
Central incisor	6-10 months	6-7 years

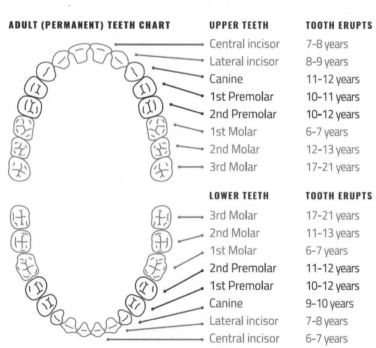

ADULT (PERMANENT) TEETH CHART

UPPER TEETH	TOOTH ERUPTS
Central incisor	7-8 years
Lateral incisor	8-9 years
Canine	11-12 years
1st Premolar	10-11 years
2nd Premolar	10-12 years
1st Molar	6-7 years
2nd Molar	12-13 years
3rd Molar	17-21 years

LOWER TEETH	TOOTH ERUPTS
3rd Molar	17-21 years
2nd Molar	11-13 years
1st Molar	6-7 years
2nd Premolar	11-12 years
1st Premolar	10-12 years
Canine	9-10 years
Lateral incisor	7-8 years
Central incisor	6-7 years

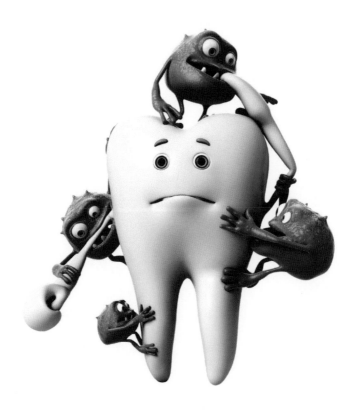

CHAPTER 2

TOOTH DECAY?

WHAT IS
TOOTH DECAY?

- Tooth decay is referred to by dentists as 'Caries.'

- 'Caries' is the softening of a tooth by acids. These acids are created by bacteria within the mouth. The bacteria creates a sticky layer, called **plaque**, which adheres to your teeth.

- When there's a lot of sugar about, these bacteria eat the sugar and produce acids as a by-product.....**that's not good!**

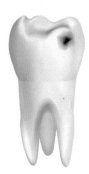 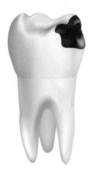 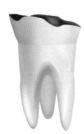

HOW DOES TOOTH DECAY PROGRESS?

1. Demineralisation

Enamel contains calcium in addition to other minerals. The acid from the bacteria within the plaque destroys these minerals. When this occurs, you may see a **white spot** appear on one of your teeth. This 'white spot lesion' is the result of calcium coming away from the enamel, and usually represents the first sign of tooth decay.

2. Breakdown of the Enamel

As caries progresses, the white spot lesion becomes darker in appearance. This results in the enamel becoming weaker which allows acid from the bacteria to further damage the teeth.

3. Breakdown of the Dentine

Once the bugs have weakened the enamel, they grow in number and progress deeper into the tooth towards the dentine. Once they reach the dentine, caries takes place at a much quicker rate.

This is because dentine is much softer than enamel making it more sensitive to the acid. By this stage, there's no turning back and **you're going to need a filling!**

4. Breakdown of the Pulp

Once those nasty bugs reach the pulp of the tooth, things get bad! The pulp is the innermost layer of your tooth. It contains all the nerves and blood vessels that keep the tooth alive. Essentially, the pulp is the 'heart' of the tooth, and once damaged, the tooth will inevitably die sooner or later.

5. Dead Tooth & Dental Abscess

When something dies, it gets **infected**, and teeth are no different. Once in the pulp, the bacteria destroy the tooth's blood vessels and nerves. This creates turmoil within the pulp resulting in the tooth dying. Left untreated, you'll end up with a pocket of pus forming at the bottom of your tooth. This is called an **abscess.**

THE 4 STAGES OF TOOTH DECAY

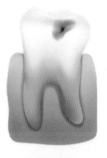

ENAMEL CARIES

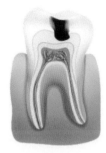

DENTINAL CARIES

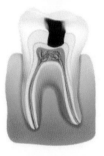

PULPAL CARIES

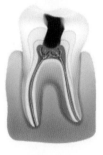

DENTAL ABSCESS

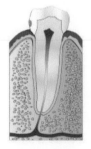

LOSS OF MINERAL

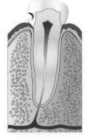

ENAMEL CARIES

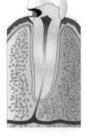

DENTINAL CARIES

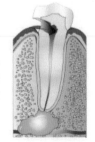

DENTAL ABSCESS

WHAT CAUSES
TOOTH DECAY?

1. Refined Carbohydrates in Food

Any food that increases the chances of us getting tooth decay is referred to as **'cariogenic food.'**

When foods rich in carbohydrates (or carbs) get trapped between teeth and are **not** completely removed by brushing or flossing, they attract nasty bugs to the area, and this is how 'caries' begins.

If you were to take a sample of these nasty bugs and look at them under a microscope, the most common one you'd see goes by the name **Streptococcus mutans (SM)**.

SM is one of the most common strains of cariogenic bacteria.

Carbs are present in a lot of food, but some carbs are more cariogenic than others.

Food that clings to your teeth are the most likely to promote tooth decay since they **attract** a lot of these SM bacteria.

Cariogenic Foods

In a nutshell, **all foods containing sugar** will significantly increase the chances of you getting tooth decay.

The most cariogenic foods out there are sweets, chocolate, and sugar-rich fruit juices.

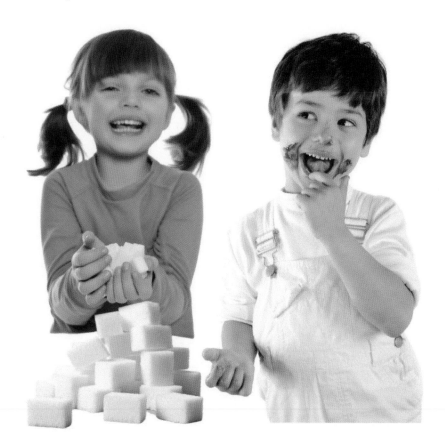

EXAMPLES OF CARIOGENIC FOODS

The table below highlights examples of foods that are associated with tooth decay.

OBVIOUS EXAMPLES OF CARIOGENIC FOODS	LESS OBVIOUS EXAMPLES OF CARIOGENIC FOODS
TABLE SUGAR	TOMATO KETCHUP
CHOCOLATES	DATES
JUICES	BANANAS
FIZZY DRINKS	MILK
SWEETS	SWEET YOGHURT
SUGAR-RICH CEREALS	WHITE PASTA
JAM	WHITE BREAD
CAKES	APRICOTS
BISCUITS	DRIED FOODS
FRUIT CANNED IN SYRUP	HONEY
BARBECUE MARINADE	FRUIT SMOOTHIES
SWEET BREAD	PASTA SAUCES
FRUIT SMOOTHIES	POTATO CHIPS

2. Frequent Snacking

Fans of intermittent fasting would love this one!!

As you surely know by now, the more often you eat during the day, the more bits of food you're likely to harbour within the mouth. Over time, this attracts more of those nasty bugs which, in turn, increases the risk of decay.

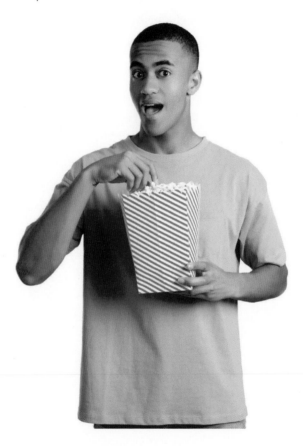

3. Eating Before Going to Bed

Saliva is a powerful **natural defence** against tooth decay. It can wash sugar out of your mouth into the stomach, fight bacteria as well as reduce the damaging effect of bacterial acids on teeth. In addition to these obvious benefits, saliva can reverse the early stages of tooth decay by repairing tooth mineral.

Therefore, if we don't produce a lot of saliva, we significantly increase the risk of tooth decay. Generally speaking, we produce **less** saliva at night. This is especially the case if one snores or breathes with their mouth open.

Having food debris in the mouth at this time feeds those nasty cariogenic bacteria. This is why night-time eating before bed is a massive no-no!

4. Poor Oral Hygiene

It's not rocket science! Plaque attaches to teeth and contains the bugs that cause tooth decay. The sugar feeds the bugs in the plaque and the damage begins thereafter!

Brushing and flossing your teeth throughout the day removes plaque and hence reduces the chance of getting tooth decay.

HOW TO PREVENT
TOOTH DECAY!

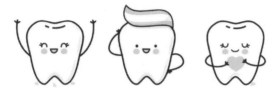

1. <u>Change Your Diet</u>

- Cut down on the amount and frequency of **Sugar-Rich Foods**

- Eat less frequently throughout the day!

- Drink lots of water and keep your mouth hydrated!

- Sugar-free chewing gum after meals is not a bad idea. Saliva is very important for protecting your teeth from decay, and chewing gum significantly boosts saliva production.

- Avoid late night eating before bed.

- Eat more 'tooth-friendly foods,' such as green vegetables, lettuce, oily fish, and so on. These foods help to protect our teeth, keep them strong, and are extremely beneficial for overall health.

Examples of Tooth-Friendly Foods

Foods that are rich in starch and sugar attract a plethora of cariogenic bacteria. When it comes to general health and well-being, our aim should be to minimise the consumption of such foods.

Now, we've already gone over the foods that are bad for our teeth, but what about the food that can make our teeth stronger?

Well, there are quite a few. I have included some examples in the table below.

TOOTH-FRIENDLY FOODS	TOOTH-FRIENDLY FOODS
BROCCOLI	BRUSSEL SPROUTS
SPINACH	KALE
CHEESE	PEAS
STRAWBERRIES	MILK
LOTS OF WATER	LETTUCE
HARD FRESH APPLES	SALMON
SEA BASS	CUCUMBER
TOFU	WALNUTS
CASHEW NUTS	BRAN

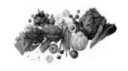

2. IMPROVE YOUR ORAL HYGIENE

- Plaque literally sticks to your teeth and harbours a plethora of nasty bugs. These bacteria contribute towards tooth decay and gum disease. The best way to fix this problem boils down to brushing and flossing your teeth on a regular basis.

- Clean between your teeth with floss or interdental brushes eg. TePe brushes.

- Drink lots of water and keep your mouth hydrated!

- Use **fluoridated toothpastes** to brush your teeth with. Fluoride kills cariogenic bacteria, helps remineralise the enamel, and aids in the prevention of tooth decay. This is the main reason why most toothpastes contain fluoride. Despite the controversy surrounding the use of fluoride, it's perfectly safe to use in moderate amounts. However, applying 'too much' fluoride over a long time period can sometimes give rise to white and brown patches around the enamel surface. This is known as 'mottled enamel.'

- All parents should brush their child's teeth until they're competent enough to do so on their own. Children under the age of 8 should use the **'children's toothpaste.'** Children over the age of 8, however, can start using the 'adult' toothpaste, but only a pea-sized amount is recommended in the beginning.

3. Visit Your Dentist Regularly

- Visit your dentist at least 1 to 2 times a year.

- The purpose of a regular check up is to allow your dentist to monitor caries-risk, oral hygiene status, and treat any potential problems before they get any worse.

- Having regular check-ups, therefore, allows your dentist to intervene early should any dental-related problems develop.

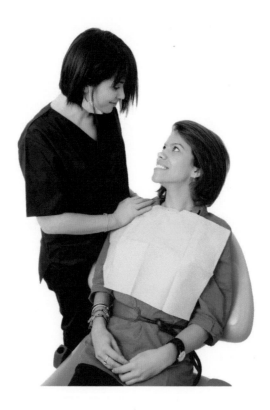

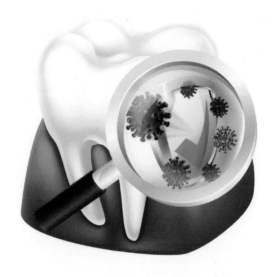

CHAPTER 3

GUM DISEASE

WHAT IS GUM DISEASE?

- A 'healthy' tooth is firm and well supported. This is because teeth are attached to the jawbone by the surrounding gums and supporting ligaments.

- 'Gum disease' occurs when these supporting tissues get infected. When this happens they may start to bleed, hurt, and swell. In severe cases, this infection and inflammation leads to the total destruction of the supporting tissues. With nothing left to support the tooth, it eventually becomes loose and drops out.

- There are 2 types of gum disease; **gingivitis** and **periodontitis**.

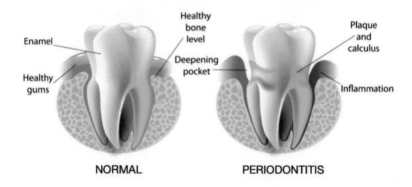

NORMAL   PERIODONTITIS

THE PROGRESSION
OF GUM DISEASE

1. <u>Normal Healthy Tooth & Gums</u>

Before we can talk about gum disease, let's see what healthy gums look like.

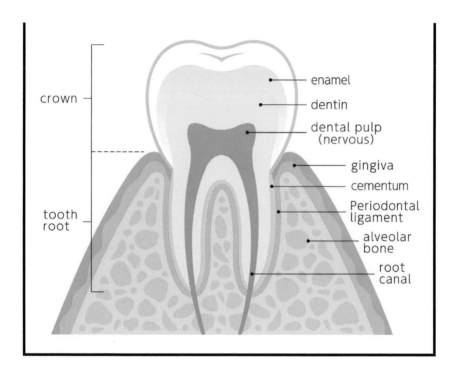

- The **alveolar bone** makes up part of the jaw bone and finishes just below the neck of the tooth.

- The **cementum** acts like the enamel of the roots. In other words, it surrounds and protects the dentine beneath the gums.

- The **periodontal ligament** is like a series of tough collagenous threads which attach the alveolar bone to the cementum. It connects the tooth to the bone.

- The **gingiva** (which is basically a fancy word for gums) covers and protects the underlying bone. It also provides a seal around the tooth. This seal prevents any bacteria within the mouth from damaging the periodontal ligament and the underlying alveolar bone.

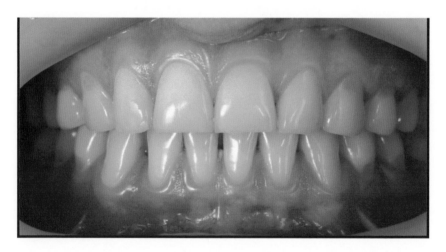

2. Gingivitis

Gingivitis can be defined as the inflammation of the gums.

It's often characterised by bleeding, red and swollen gums.

Gingivitis is the first stage of gum disease.

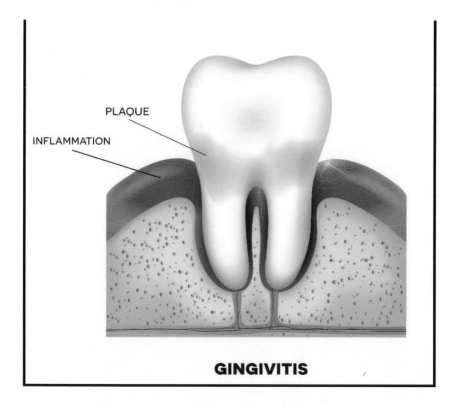

PLAQUE

INFLAMMATION

GINGIVITIS

- When you forget to brush or floss, a sticky film consisting of bacteria and food (ie. **plaque**) builds up around your teeth. This layer of plaque can cause tooth decay and infect the gums. This often results in **'gingivitis.'**

- After 72 hours, plaque solidifies into a hard substance called **'tartar.'** With time, tartar attracts more plaque to the tooth by making the teeth harder to clean. Tartar can only be properly removed by your dentist or hygienist.

- A build up of plaque can cause the gums to become red, swell, bleed, hurt, and even smell.

- Fortunately, a few visits to the dentist in addition to brushing and flossing more frequently is usually all that's needed in order to treat gingivitis.

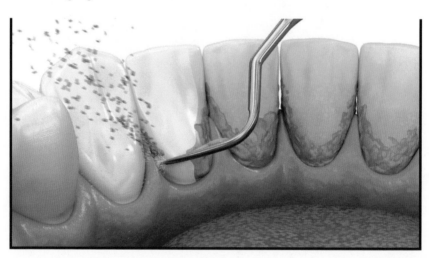

3. <u>Moderate Periodontitis</u>

Periodontitis is defined as the inflammation of the periodontal ligament.

Moderate periodontitis occurs when gingivitis is not treated in time. This results in the disease progressing from the gums to the deeper tissues.

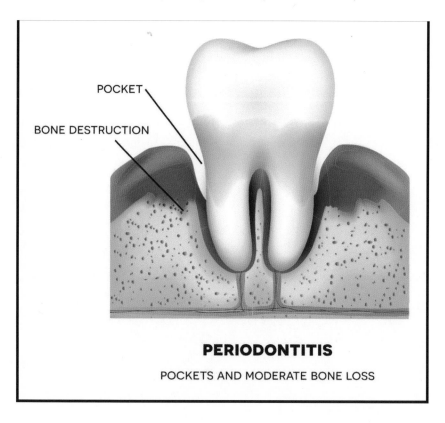

PERIODONTITIS

POCKETS AND MODERATE BONE LOSS

- Gingivitis is limited to the gums. Periodontitis, on the other hand, is the result of plaque deposits getting bigger in size and causing damage to the gum line, periodontal ligament, and alveolar bone. Therefore, the structures supporting the tooth become weakened. In some cases, this can make the tooth feel looser.

- Patients suffering from periodontitis tend to have red, swollen and tender gums. In addition, they often have bad breath, and bleed a lot whilst brushing.

- Unfortunately, periodontitis is not always reversible. However, if it's caught early and the patient is willing to drastically improve his/her oral hygiene, successful management of the disease is more likely.

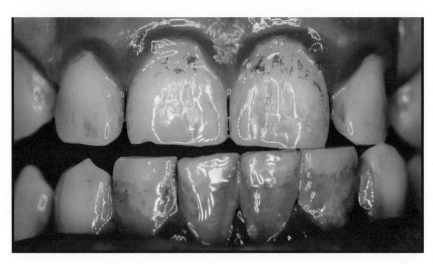

4. <u>Advanced Periodontitis</u>

This is the final stage of gum disease.

Advanced periodontitis occurs when the earlier phases of gum disease go untreated.

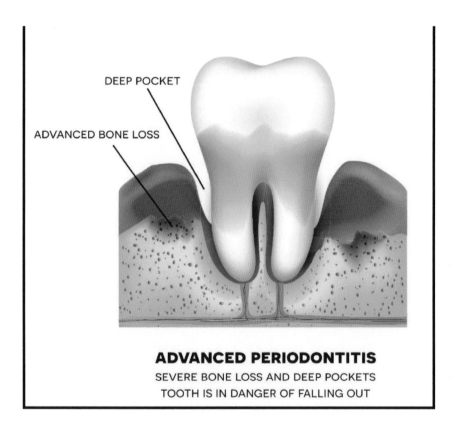

ADVANCED PERIODONTITIS
SEVERE BONE LOSS AND DEEP POCKETS
TOOTH IS IN DANGER OF FALLING OUT

- Advanced periodontitis is the third and final stage of gum disease.

- By this stage, there are a plethora of bacteria well below the gum line. This infection unfortunately creates more room for these festering bacteria to thrive. Advanced periodontitis represents the point of no return. The damage is often irreversible.

- Patients with advanced periodontitis often have swollen gums and loose teeth. In some cases, pus may escalate from the gums.

- By this stage, the bone and periodontal ligament are badly damaged. As a result, the tooth becomes very loose. In addition, it's also painful to bite on due to the pus around the roots pushing the tooth out of its socket.

- Extraction and antibiotics are the only treatment options at this point.

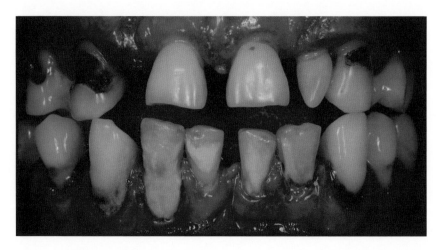

HOW TO PREVENT AND
TREAT GUM DISEASE

1. Brush Your Teeth Properly!!!

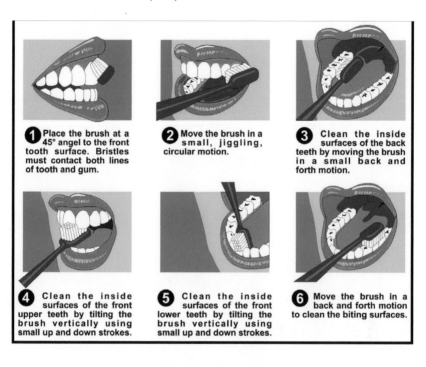

1. Place the brush at a 45° angel to the front tooth surface. Bristles must contact both lines of tooth and gum.

2. Move the brush in a small, jiggling, circular motion.

3. Clean the inside surfaces of the back teeth by moving the brush in a small back and forth motion.

4. Clean the inside surfaces of the front upper teeth by tilting the brush vertically using small up and down strokes.

5. Clean the inside surfaces of the front lower teeth by tilting the brush vertically using small up and down strokes.

6. Move the brush in a back and forth motion to clean the biting surfaces.

- Always using a **soft-to-medium bristled** toothbrush (manual or electric). Opt for using anti-cavity **fluoride-rich** toothpaste.

- When brushing, use a circular motion holding the toothbrush at 45-degrees to the gum line.

By doing this, you will be able to successfully remove plaque from the crevices between the gum margins and the teeth without damaging the gums themselves.

- The minimum length of time you should brush your teeth for is **2 minutes twice a day!** Remember to include the inside, outside, and biting surfaces of the teeth. Bacteria **also** live on your gums, tongue, and roof of your mouth (ie. your palate). Therefore, you can benefit from brushing these areas as well as your teeth.

- However, when brushing your gums and soft tissues, use very gentle pressure or **ideally a soft brush**. Avoid brushing teeth in an excessively hard manner as doing so will eventually cause your teeth to wear and your gums to recede.

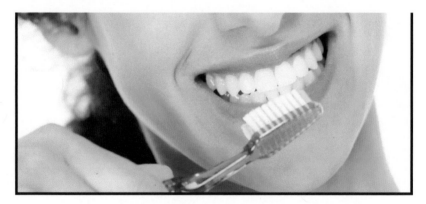

2. <u>Floss More Regularly!!</u>

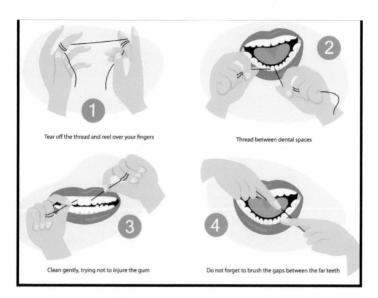

Tear off the thread and reel over your fingers

Thread between dental spaces

Clean gently, trying not to injure the gum

Do not forget to brush the gaps between the far teeth

- Flossing helps to remove food and plaque from areas of the mouth that **aren t** accessible with a normal toothbrush. In other words, the reason why we floss is to remove plaque from between and behind our teeth.

- When flossing, use a long piece of floss (around **18 inches**), wrap it around your fingers, and make a C" shape as you do it each time.

- As opposed to just going up and down, try to scrape **each surface** of the tooth. Guide the floss all the way down to your gum pockets (ie. as low as you can). **Don't worry if your gums bleed at this point**, the bleeding will lessen over time as they start to heal.

- If you don t like using conventional floss, there are alternatives you can use such as **TePe Brushes, flossettes** (or floss in a holder), and **super-floss** (which is great for cleaning around braces, bridges, etc).

- Whichever method you prefer, you should floss/clean between your teeth **at least once a day** in addition to brushing your teeth for 2 minutes.

  Aim to brush and floss your teeth two to three times a day.

3. Finish Off With A Good Mouthwash

- Once you ve flossed and brushed your teeth, there s nothing like using a good mouthwash to finish off with. In saying that, however, you should **NEVER** use a mouthwash as an **alternative** to brushing and flossing.

- A mouthwash is, rather, the proverbial icing on the cake. A **one-minute rinse** should suffice whatever mouthwash you use.

- There is no shortage of mouthwashes on the market. Therefore, it can be understandably quite difficult to decide which one to go for.

- As a general rule of thumb, I d recommend **Listerine Total Care** as a great all-round mouthwash.

- 'Colgate Plax' is an excellent, alternative to Listerine. It's ideal for patients who are looking for a less stingy, alcohol-free mouthwash.

- 'Corsodyl' and 'Corsodyl Daily' are more suited for those suffering from or prone to gum disease. The original '**Corsodyl**' mouthwash may, however, stain your teeth after a while so use in moderation.

- 'UltraDex Mouthwash' is an excellent mouthwash for those suffering from bad breath.

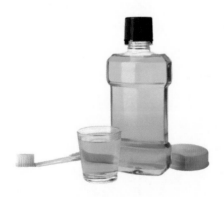

4. Boost Your Immunity

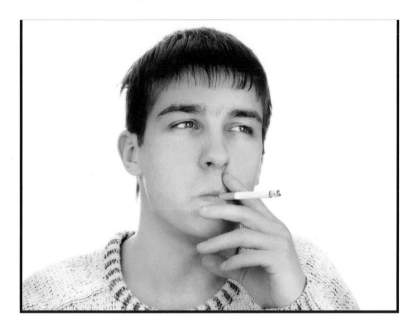

- Anything that harms your immune system increases the chances of **you** getting gum disease.

- Do the following to boost your immune system:

BOOST IMMUNE SYSTEM	BOOST IMMUNE SYSTEM
AVOID/STOP SMOKING	EAT MORE LEAFY GREENS
AVOID/REDUCE STRESS	EXERCISE REGULARLY
REDUCE STRESS	SLEEP FOR 7HRS/NIGHT

-

5. Visit Your Dentist Regularly

- Visit your dentist at least 1 to 2 times a year.

- The purpose of a regular check up is to allow your dentist to monitor caries-risk, oral hygiene status, and treat any potential problems before they get any worse.

- Having regular check-ups, therefore, allows your dentist to intervene early should any dental-related problems develop.

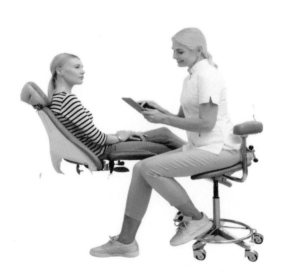

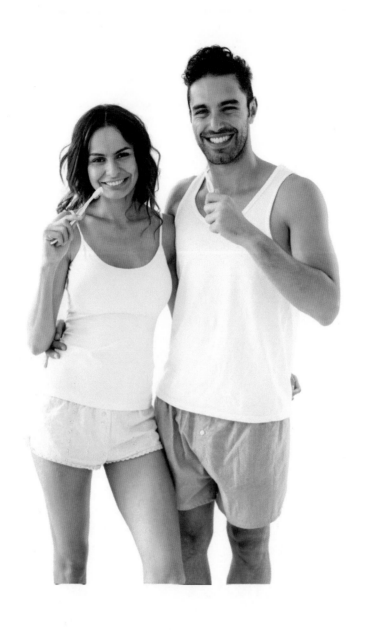

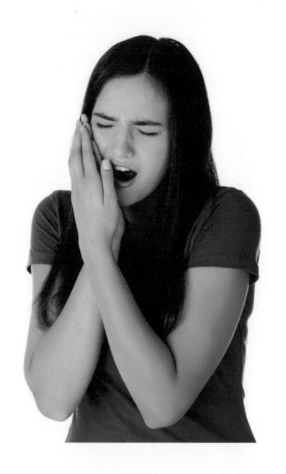

CHAPTER 4

TOOTH PAIN

COMMON CAUSES
OF TOOTHACHE

- Toothache can be one of the worst type of pain you'll ever experience. But why do we get toothache? Well, before we get into that, the list below shows the commonest reasons why we get tooth pain.

CAUSES OF TOOTH PAIN	CAUSES OF TOOTH PAIN
DENTAL ABSCESS	TRAUMA
PULPITIS	GINGIVITIS
PERIODONTITIS	BRUXISM AND TMJD
DRY SOCKET	CRACKED TOOTH SYNDROME

-

- Now this is not an exhaustive list as there are a few other causes of tooth pain which I have intentionally left out. However, the list above highlight the commonest causes.

- In this chapter, we're going to delve into how these dental disorders contribute to toothache.

WHAT THE HELL
IS PULPITIS???

- The core of a healthy tooth consists of soft, fleshy tissues comprising of nerves and blood vessels. Collectively, these tissues are referred to as the **'pulp.'**

- The pulp provides vital nutrients to the rest of the tooth. These nutrients keep the tooth moisturised, healthy, strong, and vital.

- As well as carrying out these important functions, the pulp also gives us warning signs, in the form of **pain or sensitivity**, if there's any 'trouble' brewing within or around the tooth.

- In other words, when our teeth are under attack or going through some form of physical trauma, the pulp gets inflamed. When this happens, the tooth often becomes sensitive and painful.

- This discomfort is nature's way of telling us that there's a problem and something needs to be done about it.

- This inflammation of the pulp is called **'pulpitis.'**

1. What Causes 'Pulpitis?'

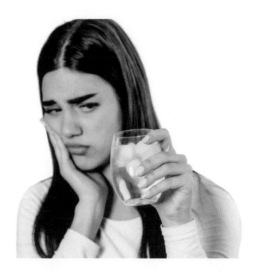

Basically, **anything** that leads to the destruction of part or all of a tooth in any way can cause pulpitis.

Tooth decay is by far the commonest cause of pulpitis, but other causes are listed below:

* **Bacterial infection** Caries/tooth decay.

* **Trauma** - Any physical injury or trauma to a tooth may cause pulpitis, even if the tooth remains intact.

* **Fractured Tooth** - Physical damage or trauma exposing the underlying dentine and/or pulp.

* **Deep Fillings & Invasive Dentistry** - Having a lot of dental work or large fillings placed into your teeth may inadvertently cause pulpitis.

* **Erosion** Exposing your teeth repeatedly to acid. Examples include fizzy drinks, fruit juice, or stomach acid such as with 'gastric reflux' or 'bulimia' cases. Acid gradually destroys your protective outer

enamel and exposes the underlying dentine and even the pulp, in severe cases. This can lead to pupitis.

- **Bruxism and Tooth Grinding** These forms of physical attrition can sometimes cause pulpitis.

- **Cracked Tooth Syndrome** is a condition whereby a tooth has incompletely cracked but no part of the tooth has yet broken off. Such tooth fractures can lead to pulpits in some cases.

2. Reversible vs Irreversible Pulpitis

- There are 2 types of pulpitis; reversible pulpitis and irreversible pulpitis.

- Reversible pulpitis represents the early phases of pulpal inflammation, whilst irreversible pulpitis represents the latter stages of pulpal inflammation.

- **Over 80 per cent of patients** who experience toothache are either going through reversible pulpitis or (more likely) irreversible pulpitis, **so we should really pay attention to this here.**

3. Tooth Decay and Pulpitis

- Because tooth decay is the commonest cause of pulpitis, we will focus on the relationship between caries progression and pulpitis.

- For the most part, tooth decay starts off in the enamel. **Enamel** is a hard, mineralised superficial layer which **doesn't** have much sensation, unlike the underlying dentine and pulp. Therefore, enamel caries is often asymptomatic. In other words, you may not suspect that you have a problem if the decay is limited to the enamel because it won't elicit pulpitis, and hence won't hurt.

- Fortunately, **enamel caries can be reversed without necessarily seeing a dentist** (although you should still see your dentist...of course).

- Modifying your diet and cleaning the carious area with a fluoridated toothpaste can successfully remineralise the enamel and eliminate further decay.

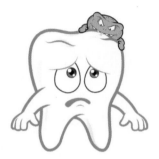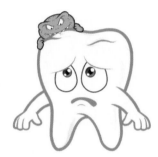

4. Reversible Pulpitis and Dentinal Caries

- Things start to get nasty once the decay progresses into dentine. When this happens, the dentine becomes exposed to air because the enamel is now weakened.

- So once the bacteria make their way into the dentine, the pulp becomes inflamed. This initial, early pulpitis is called 'reversible pulpitis.'

- **'Reversible pulpitis,'** as the name suggests, is reversible. We can, therefore, successfully treat the inflammation in most cases without harming the pulp.

- Once treated, the **pulp miraculously heals itself** and eventually function as normal.

- A filling placed by your dentist, in conjunction with an improvement in diet and oral hygiene, will treat 'reversible pulpitis' successfully in most cases.

- Reversible pulpitis is usually diagnosed by your dentist and characterised classically by the symptoms in the table below.

SYMPTOMS OF REVERSIBLE PULPITIS	
SENSITIVITY TO COLD FOOD AND DRINKS	TOOTH DOESN'T HURT WHEN TAPPED
SENSITIVITY TO SWEETS	PAIN IS SHARP AND SHORT
PAIN OR SENSITIVITY LASTS SECONDS	PAIN GOES AWAY ONCE STIMULUS IS REMOVED

·

EXAMPLES OF TOOTH DECAY SPREADING INTO DENTINE

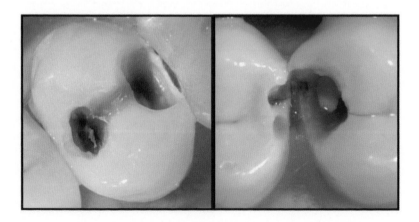

5. Irreversible Pulpitis and Deep Caries

- **Irreversible pulpits** takes place when the bacteria has already spread throughout the tooth and reached, or come very close to, the pulp.

- By this stage, the inflammation has become **irreversible** meaning the pulp has no chance of survival.

- When most parts of the body get inflamed, a noticeable swelling occurs. If you bang your finger, for instance, it may swell and becomes tender. These symptoms are classic signs of inflammation.

- When a tooth gets inflamed, however, the pain can become unbearable. Irreversible pulpits is characterised by a severely inflamed pulp. Unlike with the above example of the swollen finger, however, the pulp cannot swell in size because, unfortunately, it's trapped within 4 walls of hard dentine and enamel. When the pulp gets inflamed and tries to swell within the confinement of these 4 walls, therefore, it gives rise to an agonising, excruciating, and pulsating toothache which is often described as the **'worst pain ever'** by so many patients.

- The only treatment at this stage is either the total removal of the pulp (ie. root canal therapy), or extraction of the tooth.

SYMPTOMS OF IRREVERSIBLE PULPITIS	
INTENSE AND EXCRUCIATING PAIN	SENSITIVITY TO COLD LASTING OVER 30 SECONDS
SENSITIVITY TO HOT AND COLD	TOOTHACHE MAY START SPONTANEOUSLY
PAIN MAY SPREAD TO AND INCLUDE OTHER TEETH	PAIN IS OFTEN WORSE AT NIGHT KEEPING YOU AWAKE
THROBBING AND PULSATING PAIN	DIFFICULTY PINPOINTING WHERE PAIN IS COMING FROM

EXAMPLES OF TOOTH DECAY SPREADING INTO PULP

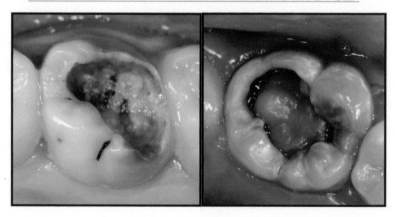

WHAT IS MEANT BY
A DENTAL ABSCESS?

- An abscessed tooth, or a **dental abscess**, is a collection of pus that can form in different parts of a tooth as a direct result of a bacterial infection.

- There are 3 main types of dental abscesses:

    - Periapical Abscess

    - Periodontal Abscess

    - Gingival Abscess

1. Periapical Abscess

- If pulpits is **not** treated in time, the pulp, and hence the tooth, will die. Once this happens, the tooth and the area around it become infected.

- The infection typically occurs around the bases of the roots, known as the 'root apex.' This is why it's called a **'periapical abscess.'**

- **In a nutshell,** a periapical abscess is a collection of pus that builds up around the root of a tooth.

SYMPTOMS OF A PERIAPICAL ABSCESS

THROBBING TOOTHACHE	PAIN RADIATES TO YOUR EAR, NECK, AND/OR JAW
TOOTH IS PAINFUL TO BITE ON	FACIAL SWELLING
SWOLLEN GUMS ESP. AROUND ABSCESSED TOOTH	MORE PAIN WHEN LYING DOWN
FEVER AND TENDER LYMPH NODES IN JAW/NECK	TOOTH IS DISCOLORED AND/OR LOOSE

EXAMPLES OF TEETH WITH PERIAPICAL ABSCESSES

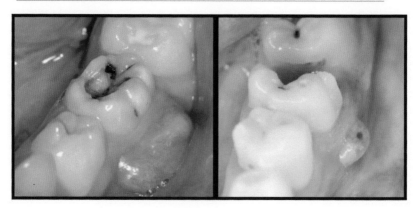

2. Periodontal Abscess

- This is an abscess on the gum next to the root of a tooth. It might also spread to the surrounding tissue and bone.

- This infection represents the final stage of 'advanced periodontitis.' In other words, a periodontal abscess is the end-result of chronic ongoing gum disease.

3. Gingival Abscess

- This is an abscess that is very similar to a periodontal abscess.

- Basically, **gingival abscesses** only occur in the gum tissue. They do not involve the teeth at all. They may occur if a sharp piece of food or debris gets lodged directly into the gums and causes an infection.

- **Periodontal abscesses,** however, occur in the space between the teeth and the gums. These are more common in people with periodontal disease, though some of these abscesses may also develop as a result of injury or food getting stuck between the teeth and the gums.

SYMPTOMS OF A PERIODONTAL AND/OR GINGIVAL ABSCESS	
A LUMP OR SWELLING WHERE THE ABSCESS IS	PUS DISCHARGE
BLEEDING GUMS	SENSITIVE TEETH AND GUMS
SHRINKING GUMS/ GUM RECESSION	LOOSE TEETH
BAD BREATH	FEVER

EXAMPLES OF PERIODONTAL AND GINGIVAL ABSCESSES

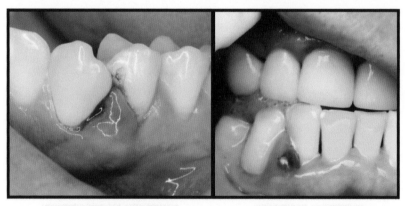

PERIODONTAL ABSCESS   GINGIVAL ABSCESS

WHAT IS FACIAL CELLULITIS??

- If a **dental abscess** remains untreated, it will likely spread to the face resulting in a facial swelling. This condition is called **facial cellulitis**.

- Facial cellulitis is an infection of the skin and underlying soft tissues, and is a potentially serious condition.

- These infections can spread very quickly. Therefore, early management is critical.

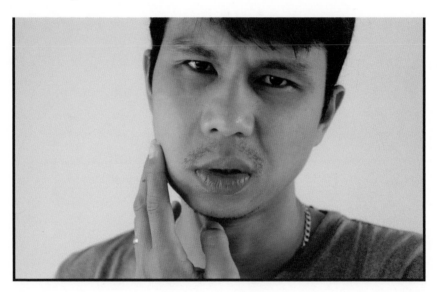

SYMPTOMS OF FACIAL CELLULITIS	
FACIAL SWELLING	PUS DISCHARGE
WEAKNESS AND LETHARGY	HEADACHE
PAIN FROM SWELLING	FEVER
LIMITED OPENING	HEADACHE

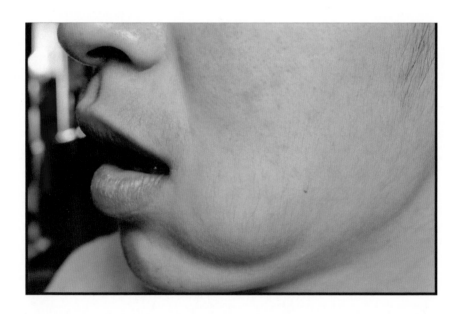

HOW TO TREAT A
DENTAL ABSCESS

- Most people with dental abscesses are initially treated with antibiotics.

- **It can take up to 2 days** before the effects of an antibiotic are noticed by the patient. The first sign of improvement, after taking a course of antibiotics, is **pain relief and a reduction in swelling.**

- Once the swelling has gone down, the tooth is often **extracted** or, at best, **root-filled.**

- A facial cellulitis is a potentially **life-threatening** complication of a dental abscess. In most cases, as with dental abscesses, oral antibiotics and subsequent visits to the dentist are usually all that's needed. Severe cases of cellulitis, however, may require hospitalisation and intravenous antibiotics.

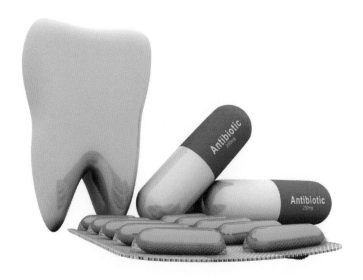

TEMPOROMANDIBULAR JOINT DISORDER (TMJD)

- This is a condition that affects the bones and muscles of the jaw.

- The **temporomandibular joint (or'TMJ')** moves your jaw whilst you re talking, eating, or even yawning. The ligaments, joints, and muscles that control your jaw are on both sides of it.

- When a misalignment occurs within these areas, or some of these muscles become overworked, your jaw experiences **stiffness and pain.**

- This set of events is collectively known as **'temporomandibular joint disorder'** or TMJD.

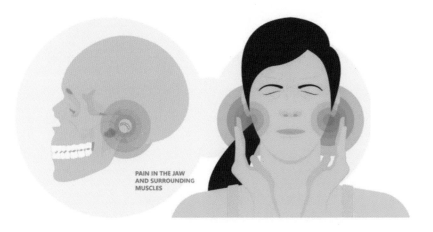

PAIN IN THE JAW AND SURROUNDING MUSCLES

1. Common Causes of TMJD

There are a number of factors that contribute towards TMJD (see below). More often than not, it is a **combination** of these factors as opposed to just one single cause.

A. Emotional Stress

Chronic stress can affect people in different ways. Some people, for instance, may consciously or subconsciously grind their teeth when they're stressed. If this becomes a common occurrence, the jaw muscles may start to become overworked, tired, tender, and painful. TMJD is a common consequence of this.

B. Bruxism

Bruxism is basically a fancy word for **'teeth grinding.'** Some patients may not be aware that they are experiencing bruxism since clenching and grinding often takes place during sleep. Night-time bruxism is a more likely cause of TMJD if the patient often finds himself/herself waking up in the morning with a stiff, painful jaw.

C. Trauma

A blow to the jaw, for example, can dislodge the joint, create localised inflammation, and potentially lead to TMJD.

D. Missing Teeth

Patients with a lot of missing teeth, especially missing back teeth, often experience TMJD. This is because the jaw muscles have to work harder in order to chew food, talk, swallow, and so on. Replacing these missing teeth with a prosthesis, such as a denture or implants, is usually all that's needed.

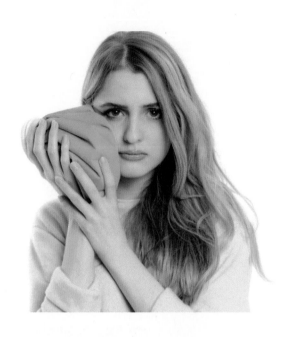

SYMPTOMS OF TMJD	
PAIN IN THE JAW AND FACIAL MUSCLES (ESPECIALLY AFTER SLEEP)	PAIN, GRINDING OR LOCKING OF THE JAW (ESPECIALLY AFTER MEALS)
HEADACHES AND DIZZINESS	CLICKING ON OPENING AND CLOSING OF MOUTH
PAIN AND DISCOMFORT WHEN YAWNING	PAIN AND DISCOMFORT WHEN TALKING/CHEWING
EAR ACHE AND SOMETIMES LOSS OF HEARING (RARE)	RINGING SOUND IN THE EARS (TINNITUS)

2. How to Manage and Treat TMJD

In most cases, the following advice is given to patients suffering with TMJD:

SOME "DO'S AND 'DONT'S"	
DO THE FOLLOWING:	AVOID THE FOLLOWING:
APPLY HEAT OR ICE FOR 15 TO 20 MINUTES ON THE AREA OF PAIN.	EXCESSIVE CHEWING (e.g. nails, gum, pen tops & your cheek).
EXERCISE YOUR JAW REGULARLY	EXCESSIVE MOUTH OPENING (e.g. yawning)
TAKE ANTI-INFLAMMATORY PAINKILLERS (eg. Nurofen)	RESTING YOUR JAW IN YOUR HAND
CHANGE TO A SOFT FOOD DIET AND AVOID HARD AND CHEWY FOODS.	HOLDING YOUR PHONE TO YOUR EARS USING JUST YOUR SHOULDERS.
CUT TOUGH FOOD INTO SMALL PIECES.	SLEEPING FACE DOWN AS THIS PUTS STRAIN ON NECK.

3. Exercise Your Jaw Regularly

- If your jaw muscles hurt when you're opening and closing your mouth, the following exercises will help things get back to normal sooner rather than later.

- Try doing these exercises a few times a day whilst taking anti-inflammatory painkillers such as nurofen.

JAW EXERCISES TO HELP TREAT TMJD

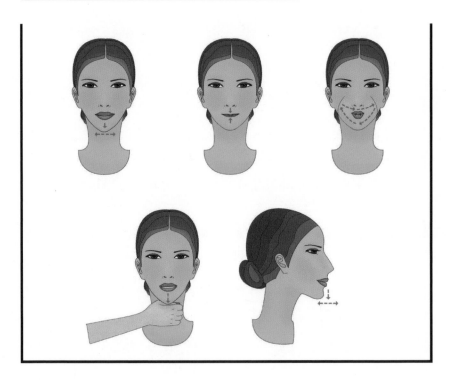

EXERCISES FOR TMJD

The following exercises are prescribed by most dentists to help treat TMJD

DO THE FOLLOWING EXERCISES:	HOW TO PERFORM THE EXERCISE
RESIST MOUTH OPENING	This involves adding pressure to your chin while closing your mouth. The first step is to place your thumbs under your chin. Next, place your index fingers between your mouth's ridge and the bottom of your chin. Lastly, use your fingers and thumbs and gently place a downwards pressure on your chin as you close your mouth
RESIST MOUTH CLOSING	You can also gently add pressure to your chin when opening your mouth. Firstly, place two fingers under your chin. Then, slowly open your mouth while also adding some gentle pressure with your fingers. Finally, hold this stance for about three to six seconds, and slowly close your mouth.
JAW SIDE-TO-SIDE	The first step is to bite down gently on your front teeth with an object that is around one-quarter inch thick. A suggestion is two popsicle sticks. However, you can use anything, really. After you have your object, move your jaw from side to side, ever so slowly. In addition, up the thickness of the object as this exercise gets easier" over time.

Exercises for TMJD

There are exercises you can do to help treat TMJD which are listed below:

DO THE FOLLOWING EXERCISES:	HOW TO PERFORM THE EXERCISE
JAW FORWARD	Get hold of an object, one-quarter inch in thickness. Hold it gently between your front teeth, and then move your jaw forward until your bottom teeth are in front of the top ones. As this becomes easier, switch the object with something thicker.
TONGUE LIFTS	This exercise involves opening and closing your mouth slowly, while still keeping your tongue touching the roof of your mouth. You can repeat the exercise several times.

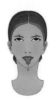 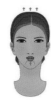 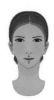

4. <u>See Your Dentist for A Splint</u>

- If the aforementioned advice doesn't work, then make an appointment to see your dentist. He/she can assess or re-assess the TMJ muscles and, if need be, make a custom-fitted plastic device, called a **splint**. A 'splint' fits over the teeth on either the top or bottom jaw. Most patients either wear the splint at night or during the day for a few hours.

- The aim of a splint is to help relax the TMJ muscles. This allows for **pain-free movement** of the jaw. Splints tend to be successful 80 per cent of the time and is often all that's needed.

- In rare cases, should this treatment not work, a referral by your dentist to an oral surgeon may be indicated for further diagnosis.

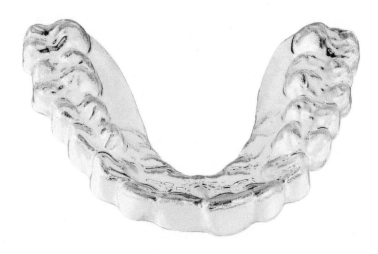

DRY SOCKET
(ALVEOLAR OSTEITIS)

"Last week, I stayed up all night in pain from toothache. The pain was so bad that I wanted to rip the tooth out myself! The next day, I made an emergency appointment to see my dentist and he took the tooth out for me. As soon as he did this, I was immensely relieved and thanked him for doing a great job. The thing is, I was so desperate for a cigarette that I didn't bother listening to the advice he gave me. Instead, I ran out of the surgery as soon as I can, went outside and lit one up. I went home that night with a numb mouth saying to myself 'I'm over the worst of it.' The next day and a few days after, however, I was still getting pain from where he took the tooth out, but this time it was even worse. I'm still in pain and now it's spread along my face. I'm in agony! Again, this has kept me up all night. For the love of God, I just want to sleep!!! Why can I not sleep???!!!"

- So that was an excerpt that a patient shared with me via social media regarding the pain he experienced before and after having an extraction.

- The description of the pain he felt after having his tooth removed are classic symptoms of a condition called **'alveolar osteitis.'** Alveolar osteitis is more commonly referred to as a **'dry socket.'**

1. What Happens After A Tooth is Pulled?

- Once your tooth has been removed, a 'hole' or tooth socket (where the tooth was) is left behind.

- This socket rapidly fills up with blood that soon forms a **blood clot**. This clot protects the hole by filling it up so that nothing in the mouth can infect the empty socket.

- The clot also protects the underlying bone and nerves within the empty tooth socket. This enables the healing process to begin. With time, new bone starts to form within the socket.

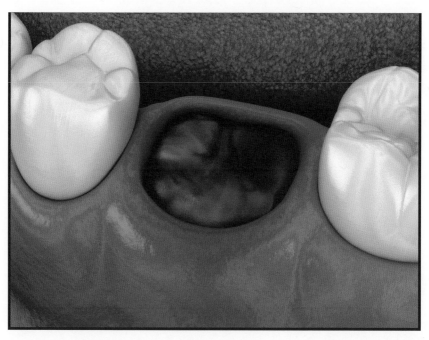

2. <u>So What Exactly is a 'Dry Socket?'</u>

- A **'dry socket'** is a condition whereby a blood clot either fails to develop, becomes dislodged, or dissolves before the wound has healed.

- This leaves the **underlying bone and nerves within the socket exposed** to the oral environment resulting in immense pain for the patient.

- To make matters worse, the socket often becomes inflamed and may fill with food debris. If you develop dry socket, the pain usually begins **one to three days** after your tooth is removed.

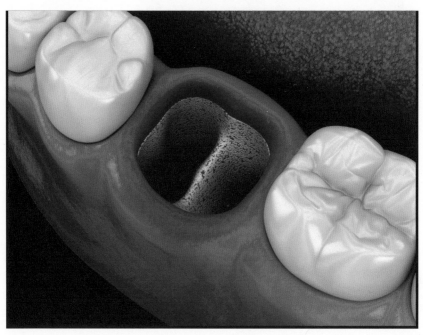

3. What Are The Symptoms of a 'Dry Socket?'

- Intense pain a day or two after a tooth extraction.

- Partial or total loss of the blood clot at the extraction site, which you may notice as an empty-looking (ie. dry) socket.

- Pain radiating from the socket to the same side of the face going as far as your eye, head or neck.

- Bad breath.

- Horrible taste.

4. What Causes a 'Dry Socket?'

We **don't know** the exact cause of dry sockets, but there are things that increase the chances of getting it. These include the following:

- Ignoring the advice given by your dentist after having the extraction.

- Smoking or tobacco products.

- Oral contraceptives.

- Bad oral hygiene.

- A history of dry socket with previous extractions.

5. How Do You Treat a 'Dry Socket?'

- Pain medication eg. Nurofen.

- Rinse with warm salty water.

- Avoid smoking.

- Apply clove oil to a sterile gauze and place over the socket.

- Apply honey to a sterile gauze and place it directly on the dry socket. Change the gauze every few hours if you keep it on consistently.

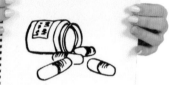

- If none of the above work, **see your dentist right away.**

- More often than not, your dentist would irrigate the area with saline and place a eugenol-based dressing called 'Alveogyl' into the socket. On occasion, a course of antibiotics would also be prescribed.

Fortunately, a dry socket only occurs in around 5% of routine tooth extractions so you'll likely be okay if you follow your dentist's advice.

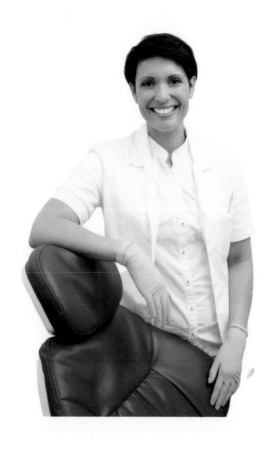

CHAPTER 5

DENTAL TREATMENT

COMMON DENTAL TREATMENTS

The most common treatments carried out in practice consist of the following:

DENTAL TREATMENT	DENTAL TREATMENT
FILLINGS	ROOT CANAL TREATMENT
CROWNS	BRIDGES
DENTURES	EXTRACTIONS
IMPLANTS	DESCALING TEETH
TEETH WHITENING	VENEERS
DENTAL SPLINTS	MOUTHGUARDS

- Now this is not an exhaustive list as there are other treatments I have intentionally not mentioned (such as botox, lip fillers, braces, Invisalign, etc.) However, the above list are by far the commonest treatments.

DENTAL
FILLINGS

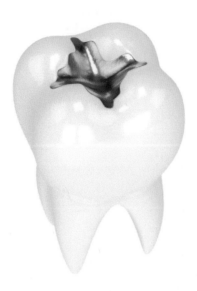

1. <u>What is a 'Filling?'</u>

- A filling is hard material that, as the name suggests, fills the hole (or cavity) remaining inside a tooth after the soft decay has been removed.

- In other words, a filling is basically a repair job to fix the damage caused by tooth decay.

- There's not a day that goes by where I don't place at least one filling into someone's tooth. This is why, out of all the dental treatments available, fillings are by far the most common.

2. <u>How Many Types of Fillings Are There?</u>

There are many types of fillings but the main ones include the following:

- **Amalgam**
  (silver fillings)

- **Composite**
  (white fillings)

- **Gold & Porcelain**
  (Inlays)

- **Glass Ionomer**
  (Temporary filling)

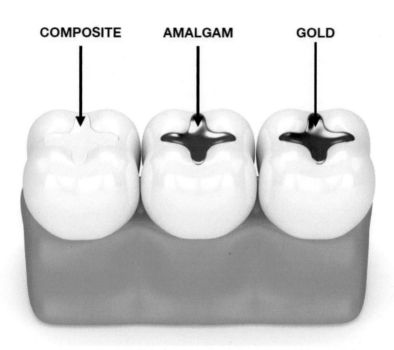

COMPOSITE   **AMALGAM**   **GOLD**

3. Which Filling Shall I Have?

Your dentist would advise which filling is best for you, but they all come with many advantages and disadvantages.

FILLING	ADVANTAGES	DISADVANTAGES
AMALGAM	DURABLE. STRONG. CHEAP. EASY TO PLACE.	UNSIGHTLY. CONTAINS MERCURY.
COMPOSITE	LOOKS GOOD. BONDS TO TOOTH. LESS DESTRUCTIVE OF TOOTH THAN AMALGAM.	MAY TAKE LONGER TO DO THAN AMALGAM. CAN BE DIFFICULT. MORE EXPENSIVE THAN AMALGAM
GOLD INLAY	DURABLE. STRONG.	EXPENSIVE. TWO VISITS (USUALLY) NEEDED.
PORCELAIN INLAY (Less common)	LOOKS GOOD. DURABLE. STRONG.	EXPENSIVE. TWO VISITS (USUALLY) NEEDED.
GLASS IONOMER FILLING (Less common)	RELEASES FLUORIDE. BONDS TO TOOTH. TOOTH-COLOURED. EASY TO USE. OFTEN USED IN CHILDREN. USED AS TEMPORARY FILLINGS.	NOT AS AESTHETIC AS COMPOSITE. VERY WEAK. SUSCEPTIBLE TO WEAR. ONLY REALLY USED AS TEMPORARY FILLINGS AND IN CHILDREN.

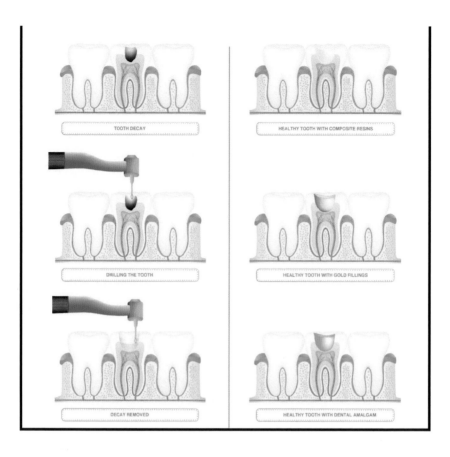

TOOTH DECAY

HEALTHY TOOTH WITH COMPOSITE RESINS

DRILLING THE TOOTH

HEALTHY TOOTH WITH GOLD FILLINGS

DECAY REMOVED

HEALTHY TOOTH WITH DENTAL AMALGAM

4. <u>What To Expect After A Filling</u>

- You will likely experience some **sensitivity to hot and cold** for a few days after. This is nothing to worry about because these symptoms usually settle within a week or two.

- However, in some cases, especially if the filling is placed close to the pulp, you may start experiencing **severe pain** a few days or weeks afterwards. This pain may well indicate irreversible pulpitis. If this happens, see your dentist right away.

ROOT CANAL
TREATMENT

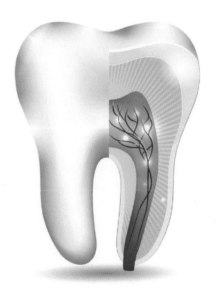

1. <u>What is a 'Root filling?'</u>

- Quite simply, a 'root filling' or 'root canal treatment' (or 'rct') is a last-resort treatment option for repairing and saving a badly damaged or infected tooth. The only alternative is to remove the tooth.

- Root canal therapy involves removing, disinfecting, and replacing the pulp of the tooth with an artificial filling material.

2. <u>What Happens During RCT?</u>

- When a tooth is **abscessed** or dying as a result of **irreversible pulpitis**, the only way of saving it is by removing the pulp. The first stage of an rct, therefore, involves the removal of the dead or dying pulp. This is achieved by using a series of **files**. Once this has been done, the now 'empty' space within the tooth is disinfected with a liquid similar to bleach.

- The dentist can then dry the canals and place a special type of filling (ie. a **'root filling'** called **'gutta percha'**) inside the disinfected empty space where the pulp, blood vessels and nerves used to be.

- The access cavity (ie. hole the dentist made in order to gain access to the pulp) is then filled with a **conventional filling eg. amalgam, composite, etc.** This filling acts like a ceiling to the underlying root filling.

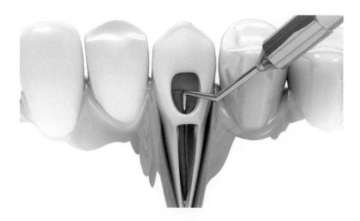

3. <u>The RCT Procedure Summarised</u>

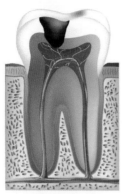

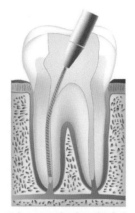

1. Toothache through
tooth decay.

2. Access to the dental pulp is
created and cleaned with instruments.

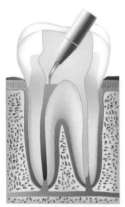

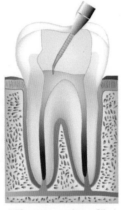

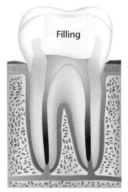

3. Rinse with antibacterial
solutions should clean and
kill bacteria.

4. The root canals are filled
with a special filling.

5. A tooth filling or a crown
sealed the tooth.

4. The Pros and Cons of RCT

- When your tooth needs an rct, the only other option is an extraction.

- So with that in mind, let's look at the pros and cons of rct versus extraction.

TREATMENT OPTION	ADVANTAGES	DISADVANTAGES
ROOT CANAL TREATMENT	SAVE/KEEP TOOTH.	DOESN T ALWAYS WORK; MAY NEED EXTRACTING IF RCT FAILS. BECAUSE RCT WEAKENS THE TOOTH, THEY OFTEN NEED TO BE CROWNED. CAN BE EXPENSIVE, ESPECIALLY IF THE TOOTH IS LATER CROWNED.
EXTRACTION	100% SUCCESSFUL. CHEAPER OPTION.	LEAVES A GAP WHERE THE TOOTH USED TO BE. FIXED REPLACEMENT OPTIONS CAN BE EXPENSIVE (eg. Bridge, Implant). DENTURES CAN BE AN UNCOMFORTABLE REPLACEMENT OPTION EXTRACTIONS CAN SOMETIMES CAUSE PAIN (eg. Dry Socket)

DENTAL
CROWNS

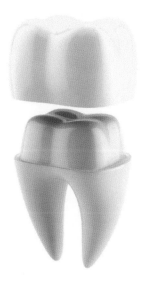

1. What is a 'Crown?'

- A 'crown' is a 'cap' that's usually placed over damaged or weakened teeth.

- In a nutshell, crowns are used to protect, cover, and restore the shape of a tooth when fillings don t solve the problem. They can also be used to improve the appearance of a discoloured tooth.

- In most cases, two or more visits to the dentist are required in order to make a crown.

2. How To Prepare A Tooth For Crowning

- On the **first visit**, the dentist undergoes a *'crown prep.'* This means the outside of the tooth is shaved circumferentially and on top by around 2mm.

- An impression of the tooth is then taken and sent off to a laboratory.

- A temporary crown is placed over the tooth in the meantime whilst the patient is waiting for the crown to be made.

- A technician uses the impressions to pour up a *working model* and make the crown before sending it back to the dentist.

- On your **second visit** to the dentist, the temporary crown is removed and the *permanent crown is cemented* to the underlying tooth.

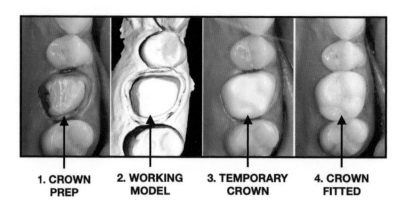

| 1. CROWN PREP | 2. WORKING MODEL | 3. TEMPORARY CROWN | 4. CROWN FITTED |

3. <u>Which Crown Should I Have?</u>

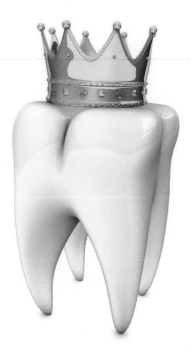

- When it comes to the types of crowns available, there are **white** ones, **silver** ones, and **gold** ones.

- In this section, I'll say a few words about each of them.

Metal Crowns

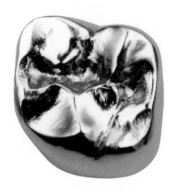

FEATURES

- METAL CROWNS ARE MADE FROM EITHER STAINLESS STEEL OR A RANGE OF METAL ALLOYS. THEY'RE STRONG IN THIN SECTIONS SO VERY LITTLE TOOTH NEEDS TO BE REMOVED IN ORDER TO ACCOMMODATE THEM.

- BECAUSE THEY ARE UNSIGHTLY, THEY'RE USUALLY PLACED OVER MOLAR TEETH SINCE THEY'RE AT THE BACK OF THE MOUTH AND ARE THEREFORE LESS NOTICEABLE.

ADVANTAGES	DISADVANTAGES
VERY STRONG.	
DURABLE.	
CONSERVATIVE OF TOOTH.	**LOOKS** *UNSIGHTLY.*
CHEAP.	

Metal Ceramic Crowns

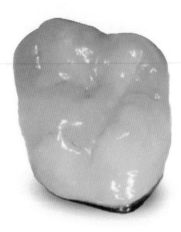

FEATURES

- THIS IS A METAL CROWN THAT HAS BEEN FUSED TO AN OUTER LAYER OF PORCELAIN FOR AESTHETICS. THIS, HOWEVER, MAKES THE CROWN THICKER MEANING MORE TOOTH NEEDS REMOVAL TO ACCOMMODATE IT.

- PORCELAIN ALONE IS VERY BRITTLE AND LIABLE TO FRACTURE, BUT THE UNDERLYING METAL SUPPORTS IT MAKING THE PORCELAIN STRONGER.

ADVANTAGES	DISADVANTAGES
MORE AESTHETIC THAN METAL CROWNS SINCE TOOTH-COLOURED.	NOT CONSERVATIVE OF TOOTH.
CAN BE USED FOR FRONT AND BACK TEETH.	NOT AS AESTHETIC AS MORE MODERN WHITE CROWNS.
OFTEN CHEAPER THAN MORE MODERN WHITE CROWNS.	PORCELAIN CAN SOMETIMES CHIP/FRACTURE EXPOSING UNDERLYING METAL.

Zirconia

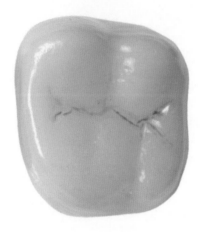

FEATURES

- ZIRCONIA IS A METAL OXIDE BUT IT'S ALSO A CERAMIC. THAT MEANS THAT IT'S EXTREMELY STRONG LIKE METAL CROWNS, BUT CONTAINS NO VISIBLE METAL AT ALL.

- THEY ARE POPULAR ALTERNATIVES TO METAL CERAMIC CROWNS BUT THEIR HEAVY DENSITY SOMETIMES MAKES THEM LESS ATTRACTIVE.

ADVANTAGES	DISADVANTAGES
MORE AESTHETIC THAN *METAL CROWNS SINCE TOOTH-COLOURED* **CAN BE USED FOR FRONT** *AND BACK TEETH.* *VERY VERY STRONG, RESILIENT TO WEAR AND DIFFICULT TO CRACK.*	**NOT AS AESTHETIC AS MORE MODERN WHITE CROWNS LIKE E-MAX FOR INSTANCE.** *EXPENSIVE.*

Emax Crowns

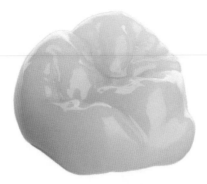

FEATURES

- EMAX IS MADE UP OF SOMETHING CALLED 'DISILICATE GLASS.' THAT BASICALLY MEANS THEY'RE VERY TRANSLUCENT AND LOOK ABSOLUTELY FANTASTIC!!

- THE PROBLEM WITH EMAX, HOWEVER, IS THAT THEY LACK THE STRENGTH OF ZIRCONIA.

- MORE RECENTLY, ZIRCONIA HAS BEEN USED UNDERNEATH EMAX TO PRODUCE A CROWN WITH EXCELLENT STRENGTH AND SUPERB AESTHETICS.

ADVANTAGES	DISADVANTAGES
SUPERB AESTHETICS. **CAN BE USED FOR FRONT AND BACK TEETH.** **RELATIVELY CONSERVATIVE OF TOOTH STRUCTURE.** *CAN BE USED WITH ZIRCONIA TO INCREASE ITS STRENGTH.*	*NOT AS STRONG AS ZIRCONIA.* *EXPENSIVE.* **EMAX CROWNS CAN** *SOMETIMES CHIP/FRACTURE, ESPECIALLY IF NOT SUPPORTED WITH ZIRCONIA.*

Full Gold Crowns

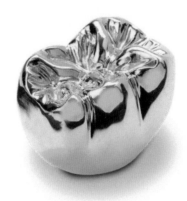

FEATURES

- TECHNICALLY, GOLD CROWNS FALL UNDER THE CATEGORY OF 'METAL CROWNS' SINCE THEY'RE NEVER 100% GOLD.

- GOLD ON ITS OWN IS TOO WEAK. THE GOLD IN GOLD CROWNS IS COMBINED WITH PALLADIUM, NICKEL, OR CHROMIUM FOR STRENGTH.

- A 'GOLD' CROWN ACTUALLY CONTAINS APPROXIMATELY BETWEEN 20% AND 60% GOLD. THE 60% GOLD CROWNS LOOK THE BEST.

ADVANTAGES	DISADVANTAGES
EXTREMELY DURABLE. **RELIABLE. THEY'VE BEEN USED IN DENTISTRY FOR OVER 4000 YEARS!** **CONSERVATIVE OF TOOTH STRUCTURE SINCE STRONG** *IN THIN SECTIONS.*	*VERY EXPENSIVE.* **IT'S NOT EVERYBODY'S CUP OF TEA FROM AN** *AESTHETIC POINT OF VIEW.*

4. When to Crown a Tooth

- The function of a crown is to help strengthen badly broken down or weakened teeth.

- Nowadays, they're also used to improve one's smile or aesthetic profile.

WHEN TO CROWN	REASON WHY
ROOT CANAL TREATED TEETH	ROOT FILLED TEETH HAVE NO PULP ANYMORE. THIS RESULTS IN A TOOTH THAT'S LIFELESS AND BRITTLE. THIS IS ESPECIALLY THE CASE WITH MOLARS AND PREMOLAR TEETH.
DISCOLORED TEETH	ALTHOUGH THERE ARE A FEW MORE 'CONSERVATIVE' MEANS OF ADDRESSING DISCOLOURATION, CROWNING IS BECOMING MORE POPULAR THESE DAYS, ESPECIALLY WITH EMAX CROWNS.
BADLY BROKEN DOWN OR HEAVILY FILLED TEETH.	IF A TOOTH MAINLY CONSISTS OF FILLING, THERE'S A MUCH HIGHER CHANCE IT WILL CHIP OR FRACTURE AFTER A WHILE. CROWNING THE TOOTH REDUCES THE CHANCE OF THIS HAPPENING.

-

A Few 'Before' and 'Afters'

- Here's a patient who's had crowns in order to fix, strengthen and mask his underlying teeth.

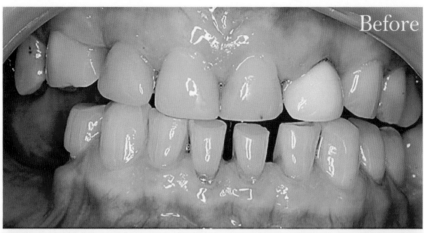

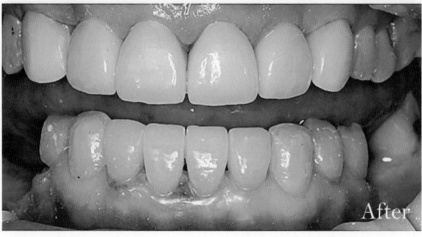

DENTAL
VENEERS

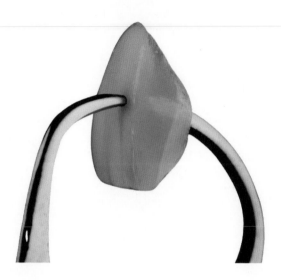

1. What is a 'Veneer?'

- A 'dental veneer' is a thin, tooth-coloured shell that's attached to the front surface of a tooth in order to improve its appearance.

- Porcelain veneers are **very similar** to crowns, but **instead** of wrapping around the entire tooth surface, veneers only cover the front and side surfaces.

2. Porcelain Veneers vs Composite Bonding

- Veneers are either **porcelain** or **composite.**

- When talking about veneers, we're usually referring to porcelain veneers. The process of making composite veneers, however, has been recently nicknamed '**Composite Bonding.**'

- The table below highlights the pros and cons of **porcelain veneers vs composite bonding.**

TYPE OF VENEER	ADVANTAGES	DISADVANTAGES
PORCELAIN VENEERS	PORCELAIN VENEERS LAST AROUND 10-15 YEARS. DUE TO THE TRANSLUCENCY OF PORCELAIN, THEY HAVE EXCELLENT AESTHETICS. PORCELAIN VENEERS ARE STAIN RESISTANT.	USUALLY REQUIRES 2 DENTAL VISITS. PORCELAIN VENEERS CAN SOMETIMES CHIP OFF OR FRACTURE. IF IT FRACTURES, THE PORCELAIN WOULD NEED REPLACING. EXPENSIVE
COMPOSITE BONDING	COMPOSITE BONDING IS USUALLY DONE IN 1 VISIT IN THE DENTIST'S CHAIR. USUALLY CHEAPER THAN PORCELAIN VENEERS. IF IT FRACTURES, CAN BE EASILY REPAIRED. COMPOSITE VENEERS ARE OFTEN REVERSIBLE SO IF YOU DON'T LIKE THEM, YOU CAN HAVE THEM REMOVED.	COMPOSITE VENEERS LAST AROUND 4 TO 8 YEARS. NOT AS STRONG AS PORCELAIN ONCE BONDED TO TOOTH. COMPOSITE IS PRONE TO STAINING OVER TIME. OFTEN NOT AS AESTHETIC AS PORCELAIN AND REQUIRES AN EXTREMELY SKILLED CLINICIAN FOR OPTIMAL RESULTS.

3. Porcelain Veneers vs Emax Crowns

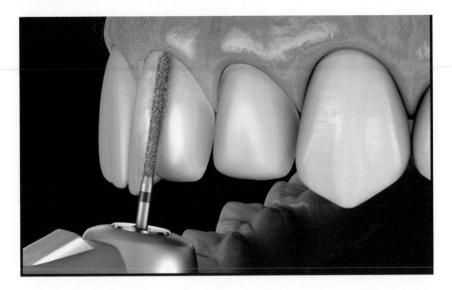

- Both porcelain veneers and Emax crowns provide superb aesthetics to the patient.

- The only real difference between porcelain veneers and (Emax) crowns is that veneers are limited to the front of the tooth/teeth. Veneers therefore **conserve** so much more natural tooth structure.

- In fact, the best results for porcelain veneers come when they're bonded to the **enamel** on the outside of the tooth. Therefore, only a small amount of tooth (0.5mm to 1mm) needs to be removed in order to prep for porcelain veneers.

4. When To Consider Veneers

Veneers are ideal in the following situations:

- Discolouration that can't be fixed with teeth whitening.

- Gaps between teeth (diastemas).

- Smaller than average teeth.

- Pointed or strangely shaped teeth.

- Teeth that are minimally restored.

- Discoloured or stained teeth with sufficient enamel.

5. When To Consider Crowns

Crowns often last longer and are preferred to veneers in the following situations:

- Heavily broken down teeth.

- Teeth that are prone to decay. Crowns cover the whole tooth which minimises risk of decay.

- Heavily filled or restored teeth.

- Eroded or worn down teeth.

- Patients who undergo a lot of contact sports.

DENTAL BRIDGES

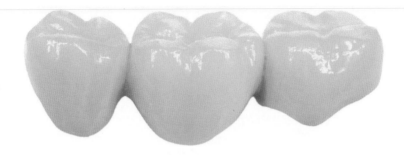

1. <u>What is a 'Bridge?'</u>

- A **'dental bridge'** is a false tooth held in place by either one or both of the teeth or implants on either side of the gap.

- Out of the 4 types of bridges available, the **'traditional conventional bridges'** and the **'conventional cantilever bridges'** are by far the commonest ones made in dental practices.

2. How Many Types of Bridges Are There?

There are **4 main types** of bridges:

TRADITIONAL CONVENTIONAL BRIDGE

A traditional dental bridge consists of a false tooth/teeth being held in place by dental crowns that have been cemented onto each of the abutment teeth.

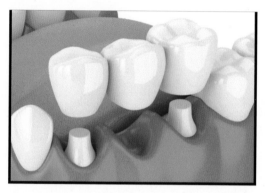

CONVENTIONAL CANTILEVER BRIDGE

A cantilever bridge is like a traditional bridge, but instead of being supported by two teeth, the bridge is supported by just one tooth.

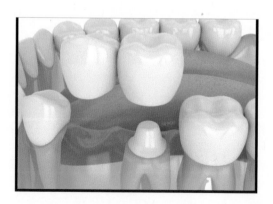

MARYLAND BRIDGE

Maryland bridges are similar to the traditional bridges but instead of the abutment tooth/teeth being crowned, a framework of either metal or porcelain is bonded onto the backs of the abutment teeth

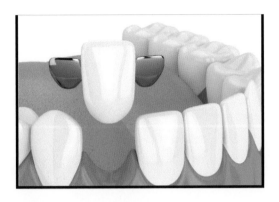

IMPLANT-SUPPORTED DENTAL BRIDGE

Implants are like screws used to replace missing teeth. These implants are usually strong enough to support at least one additional fake tooth or bridge unit.

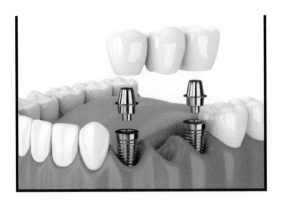

3. How To Prepare A Tooth for Bridging

Bridges can be supported by one or more teeth.

Preparing a tooth/teeth for a bridge follows a similar process to that of a crown prep.

The procedure for a **traditional** bridge prep is as follows:

- On the <u>first visit</u>, the dentist undergoes a *'bridge prep.'* This means the outside of the tooth is shaved circumferentially and on top by around 2mm.

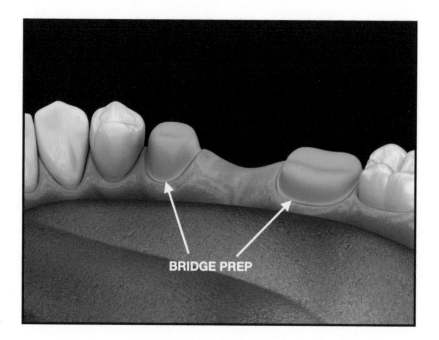

4. Fitting The Bridge After Prep

- An impression of the tooth/teeth is then taken and sent off to a laboratory. A temporary crown or bridge is placed over the tooth/teeth in the meantime whilst the patient is waiting for the bridge to be made.

- A technician uses the impressions to pour up a **working model** and make the bridge before sending it back to the dentist.

- On the <u>second visit</u> to the dentist, the temporary crown(s) or bridge is removed so that the **permanent bridge can be cemented** to the underlying tooth/teeth.

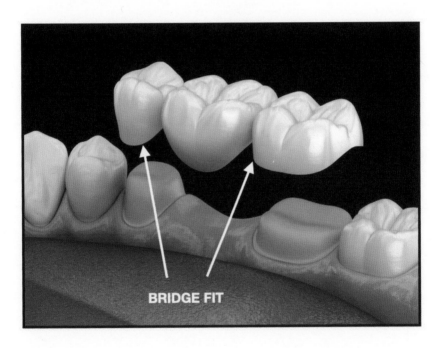

BRIDGE FIT

DENTAL
IMPLANTS

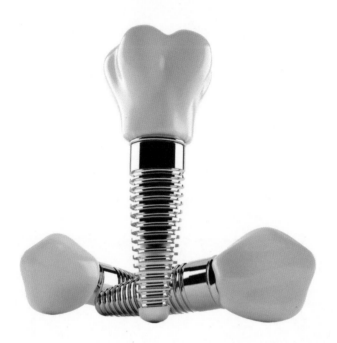

1. <u>What is an 'Implant?'</u>

- A **'dental implant'** is a metal post that replaces the root of a missing tooth. The metal is usually serrated and made of **titanium**.

- Dental implants are sometimes known as **screw-in teeth**. Implants replace missing teeth via the placement of a small titanium insert into the jawbone. They look, feel, and function like your natural teeth.

2. Implant-Retained Prosthesis

- Although we refer to these 'screw in teeth' as 'implants,' it's important to remember that an 'implant' is just the 'root' part of the prosthesis.

- In other words, an implant is a hollowed-out piece of **titanium** that's literally **screwed** into the jawbone by the dentist. Over the next month or 2, because titanium is inert, the alveolar bone literally grows into the grooves of the implant. This serves to anchor it in place.

- The function of the implant is to support crowns, bridges, and removable dentures.

- There are actually 3 components that make up a 'screw-in tooth.' and this **3-piece unit** is called an **'implant-retained prosthesis.'**

- So this '3-piece unit' consists of an implant, abutment, and prosthesis:

    a) **Implant** which acts as a root that's anchored deep within the jawbone.

    b) **Abutment** which is a piece of metal that's screwed into the inside of the implant.

    c) **Prosthesis** (ie. the crown, bridge, or denture).

3. Implant-Retained Crown

- When you have a single tooth missing, an implant-retained crown is the next best thing to having an actual tooth present.

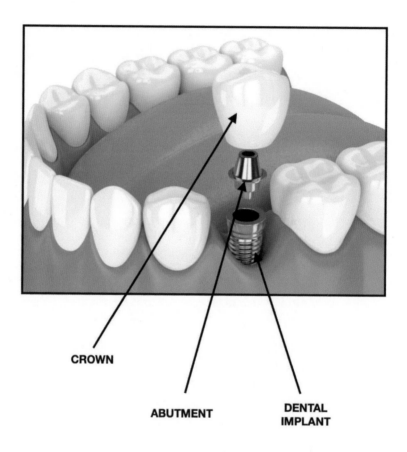

CROWN

ABUTMENT

DENTAL IMPLANT

4. Implant-Retained Bridge

- When you have 2 or more teeth missing in a row, implant-retained bridges are an excellent option.

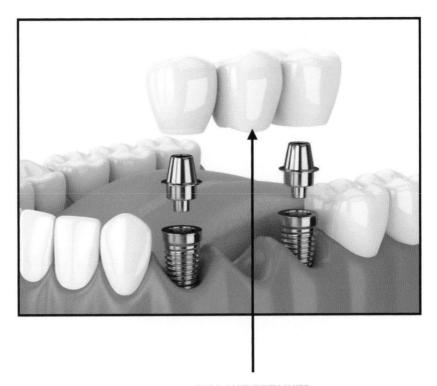

**IMPLANT-RETAINED
DENTAL BRIDGE**

5. Implant-Retained Denture

- This is a popular option for those with quite a few teeth missing or those already used to wearing a denture.

- These are essentially teeth that you can remove but are secured in the mouth with implants.

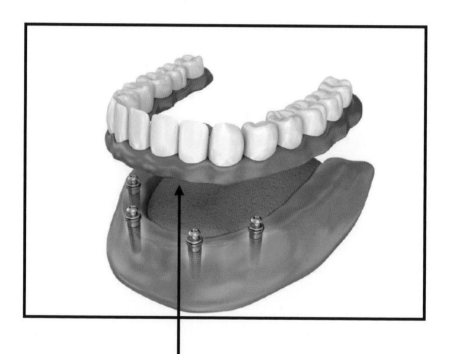

**REMOVEABLE IMPLANT-
RETAINED DENTURE**

6. <u>All-on-4 Implant-Retained Bridge</u>

- This is an excellent choice for patients with no teeth (often on the top jaw) who are looking for a fixed replacement (ie. an alternative to removable teeth).

- These teeth are literally screwed to the bone via the abutments.

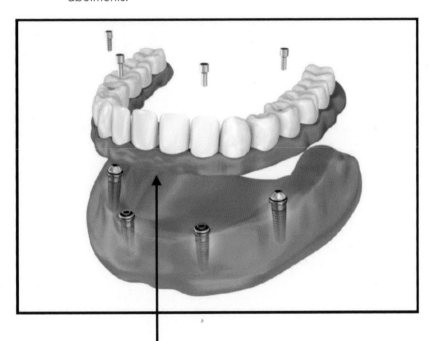

**FIXED IMPLANT-
RETAINED BRIDGE**

DENTURES

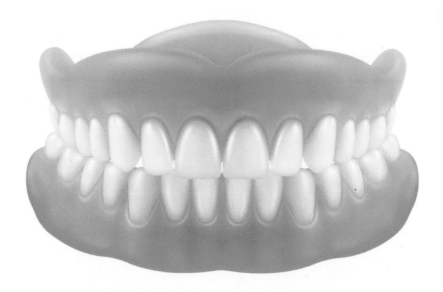

1. What is a 'Denture?'

- Dentures are removable teeth which are often referred to as 'false teeth.'

- They fit snugly over the gums to replace missing teeth and eliminate potential problems caused by gaps.

2. Types of Dentures

- Dentures are either **'complete'** or **'partial'** dentures.

- They are made out of **acrylic (plastic), nylon, or metal.**

3. Complete Dentures

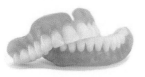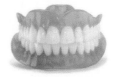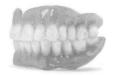

- 'Complete' or 'full' dentures are removable false teeth used to replace a full set of missing teeth.

- The **most common** type of complete denture is one made **entirely out of acrylic (plastic)**.

- However, some full dentures have a chrome (metal) base.

4. Partial Dentures

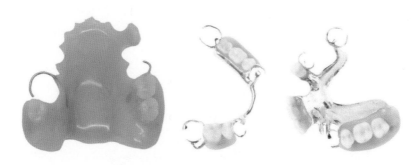

- Partial dentures are removable false teeth **designed to fill in the gaps left by one or more missing teeth**. Most partial dentures are either **acrylic, nylon (Valplast) or chrome (metal)**.

5. Acrylic Partial Dentures

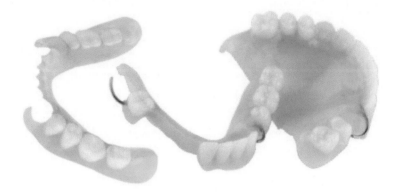

- Acrylic partials **consist of denture teeth attached to an acrylic base plate**. The denture stays in place by fitting closely and tightly against the gums and natural teeth. Sometimes, **clasps (or metal grips)** are used to provide additional retention.

6. Chrome Partial Dentures

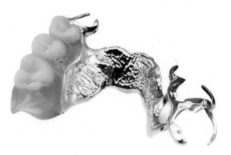

- Chromes have a **metal framework** which support acrylic teeth. They're *very thin,* and the upper ones only partly cover the palate. This makes them more comfortable (albeit **more expensive**) than acrylics.

7. Valplast Partial Dentures

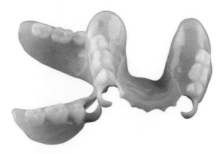

- Valplast partials are made up of a nylon resin material that's **thinner and more durable** than acrylic dentures. They are sometimes called **'Flexi'** dentures because they're bendable. Valplasts are relatively newer and very popular alternatives to acrylics and chromes.

TEETH
WHITENING

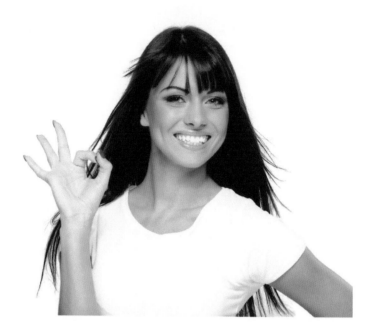

1. <u>What is 'Tooth Whitening?'</u>

- 'Tooth whitening,' sometimes referred to as **'bleaching,'** is the process of lightening the colour of your teeth.

- This process is carried out by applying a bleaching agent directly onto the teeth.

2. <u>So Why Are My Teeth Yellow??!!</u>

- Teeth discolour for a number of reasons. As you get **older**, your teeth tend to get darker and yellower anyway, but there are other reasons behind tooth discolouration.

- Some of these reasons have already been discussed. The most **common** reasons and treatments are listed below.

CAUSE	REASON	TREATMENT
TOOTH DECAY	DECAY MAKES THE TOOTH GO BLACK.	WHITE FILLING, CROWN, VENEER.
EROSION/ TOOTH WEAR	AS ENAMEL BECOMES THINNER, THE YELLOW DENTINE BECOMES MORE VISIBLE.	BLEACHING, WHITE FILLING, CROWN, VENEER.
AGE	ENAMEL OFTEN GETS THINNER & MORE STAINED AS WE AGE.	BLEACHING, VENEERS.
PLAQUE/ POOR ORAL HYGIENE (OH)	PLAQUE & FOOD STAINS DEVELOP FROM POOR OH.	IMPROVE ORAL HYGIENE, SEE A HYGIENIST.
EXTRINSIC STAINS	STAINS ON THE OUTSIDE OF TEETH.	HYGIENIST, WHITENING TOOTHPASTE.
INTRINSIC STAINS	STAINS ON THE INSIDE OF TEETH.	BLEACHING, VENEERS, CROWNS.

3. Extrinsic Staining

- These stains are caused by something that comes into contact with your teeth.

- Poor oral hygiene, tea, coffee, red wine, fizzy drinks, curries, smoking, and drugs are common causes of **extrinsic teeth staining**.

- Put simply, **anything that can stain your clothes can also stain your teeth**. Dark-coloured, pigment-rich foods that stick to enamel may cause them to appear darker and yellow.

- **Acidic foods and drinks** may erode enamel and make it even easier for stain-inducing pigments to attach to the teeth.

- Extrinsic stains can often be removed by your **dentist or hygienist**. In less severe cases, a **whitening toothpaste** alone would suffice.

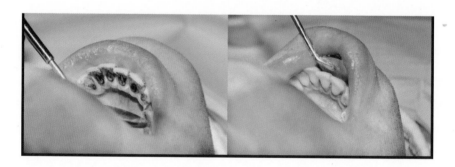

4. Intrinsic Staining

- Intrinsic stains are those that **cannot** be removed through mechanical measures such as brushing or professional cleaning. In other words, the staining comes from **within** the tooth or body.

- Common causes of 'intrinsic staining' include **ageing, tooth wear, and certain medications** such as antibiotics (eg. doxicycline, tetracycline, antihistamines).

- Other causes include **fluorosis**, and developmental problems like **enamel hypoplasia** (ie. when a patient is born with thin enamel).

- When it comes to whitening these teeth, and hence removing 'intrinsic stains,' the **only** treatment options are **bleaching, veneers, composite bonding, and crowns.**

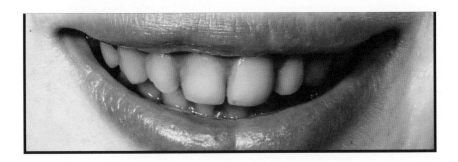

5. How To Reduce Teeth Staining

Now that we know what causes staining, we can do things to reduce it. Following the advice below will keep your teeth bright and white:

1) Rinse your mouth out with water and ideally brush your teeth before and after consuming the following:

   - Coffee
   - Tea
   - Fruit Juice
   - Blueberries
   - Beets
   - Tomato sauce
   - Soy sauce
   - Curries
   - Cola
   - Red wine

2) Use a **straw** to consume drinks.

3) Chew **sugar-free gum**; this can help to stimulate more saliva, which cleanses your mouth.

4) Brush your teeth 2 or more times a day.

5) Visit your dentist regularly.

6) Eat **more crunchy fruits and vegetables**, like apples, carrots and celery. These foods boost saliva production and scrub your teeth by becoming 'natural stain removers.'

6. How Does Teeth Whitening Work?

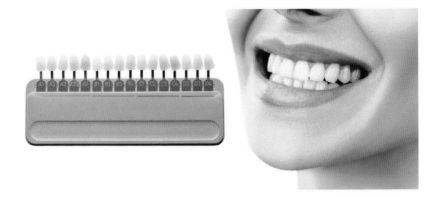

- Teeth contain certain molecules within their enamel and dentine. These molecules reflect light in a way which gives rise to the colour of your teeth.

- The bigger and more complex these molecules become, the more light they reflect and the more stained and discoloured they appear.

- Conversely, if these molecules were **smaller**, they would reflect less light. This would result in whiter teeth.

- The active ingredient in bleaching gels is **'hydrogen peroxide.'** The peroxide reacts with the large molecules within the tooth and breaks them down to small molecules. As a result, the teeth become whiter.

7. Home Bleaching

- The **best and most predictable** means of bleaching teeth involves having your dentist make custom-fitted **'bleaching trays'** in addition to prescribing **14-days worth of 'bleaching syringes.'**

- In UK, these 'bleaching syringes' usually contain either hydrogen peroxide or carbamide peroxide.

  - 6% Hydrogen Peroxide,

  - 10% Carbamide Peroxide, or

  - 16% Carbamide Peroxide.

6% Hydrogen Peroxide (Day Bleaching)

- Hydrogen peroxide works best after 30 to 60 minutes, but is not that effective after 90 minutes.

- Gels containing hydrogen peroxide are, therefore, great for people who want to bleach their teeth with minimum wear time.

- You typically only need to wear the trays for around **an hour and a half each day.**

- These gels are perfect for those who don t want to wear their trays overnight.

Carbamide Peroxide (Night Bleaching)

- Carbamide peroxide gels (CP) actually contain hydrogen peroxide, but the CP slows down and rations out its release.

- In other words, CP bleaches your teeth for **longer** than the hydrogen peroxide does **(up to 6 hours)** but is most effective around the **2-hour mark.**

- These gels are perfect for those who prefer wearing their trays whilst sleeping.

- CP is sold as 10% or 16%. A common side effect of bleaching is short-term tooth sensitivity. If you have sensitive teeth, 10% CP is recommended. If not, 16% CP is often preferred. Since the 16% CP is stronger, you'd get quicker results with 16% as opposed to 10%.

The Bottom Line

- Both hydrogen peroxide and carbamide peroxide gels work, and they'll both whiten your teeth!! The overall treatment can take between **2-6 weeks** depending on the colour of the teeth at the beginning of the treatment. In a handful of cases, however, teeth whitening **may take longer than 6 weeks.**

8. Power Bleaching

- **Power bleaching** or 'in-office' bleaching is good for those who want immediate results.

- Basically, this involves lying down in your dentist's surgery and having him/her apply a strong dose of hydrogen peroxide gel to your teeth.

- The gel is left in contact with the patient's teeth for around **15 minutes,** then removed and re-applied. **This cycle continues 4 times.**

- 'Power' whitening involves the use of a light which shines on the teeth in order to enhance the process. Power bleaching does work, but is often supplemented with home bleaching kits, and can prove to be quite expensive.

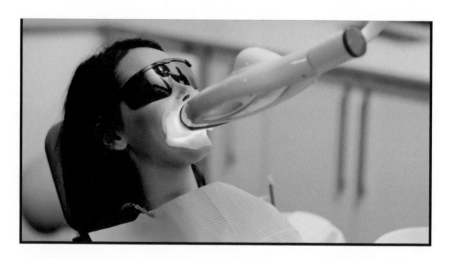

9. Frequently Asked Questions About Bleaching

QUESTION	ANSWER
WHY SHOULD I PAY MY DENTIST £300 WHEN I CAN GET BLEACHING KIT ONLINE FOR £30?????	SIMPLE. THE ONLINE STUFF IS NOT AS EFFECTIVE OR AS STRONG AS THE GELS THAT ONLY DENTISTS CAN LEGALLY USE.
IS BLEACHING HARMFUL TO YOUR TEETH?	BLEACHING IS GENERALLY CONSIDERED SAFE, AS LONG AS IT'S UNDERTAKEN BY A DENTAL PROFESSIONAL.
I HEARD BLEACHING MAKES YOUR TEETH HURT. IS THAT TRUE?	BLEACHING WILL CAUSE SHORT TERM SENSITIVITY IN MOST PATIENTS. HOWEVER, THIS SHOULDN'T LAST MORE THAN A DAY OR SO.
IS THERE ANYTHING I CAN DO TO REDUCE TOOTH SENSITIVITY?	IT'S ADVISED THAT YOU START USING AN ANTI-SENSITIVITY TOOTHPASTE LIKE 'COLGATE SENSITIVE' OR 'SENSODYNE' FOR A FEW WEEKS.
IS HOME BLEACHING AS EFFECTIVE AS POWER BLEACHING?	YES IT IS. IN FACT SOME ARGUE IT'S BETTER. HOME BLEACHING ALLOWS YOU TO APPLY THE GEL OVER A LONGER TIME PERIOD.
WILL MY TEETH BECOME YELLOW AGAIN?	THEY'RE LESS LIKELY TO DARKEN IF YOU TAKE THE STEPS MENTIONED EARLIER TO REDUCE STAINING.
DO I NEED TOP UPS?	ONCE YOU ATTAIN A DESIRED SHADE, IT'S ADVISED TO BLEACH FOR AROUND 1 WEEK A YEAR.
DO WHITENING TOOTHPASTES WORK?	WELL THEY'RE QUITE ABRASIVE SO THEY'RE NOT BAD FOR HELPING REMOVE EXTRINSIC STAINS, BUT THAT'S ABOUT IT.

DENTAL
SPLINT

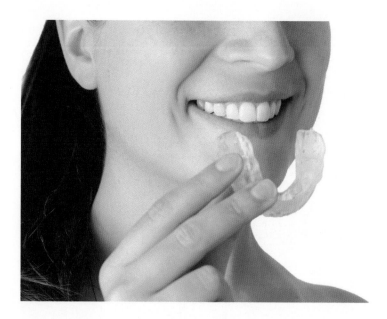

1. What is an 'Acrylic Splint?'

- A **dental splint** (or **'acrylic' splint**) is an appliance used to protect teeth and their supporting structures from damage caused by grinding or clenching.

- They work by distributing the forces generated by **bruxism** (ie. grinding and clenching) equally between the upper and lower teeth. **This reduces muscle strain and joint overloading. It also protects the teeth from further potential damage.**

2. A Few Words About Bruxism

- Bruxism is usually brought about by **stress**. Other less common causes include high-spots on fillings, over- erupted or malpositioned-teeth. Drug-use, such as cocaine, can also contribute to bruxism.

- 20% adults are aware they're grinding their teeth, and do so during the day. A smaller number of people grind their teeth whilst sleeping.

- Interestingly enough, **night-time grinders** often exert a lot more force onto their teeth (**up to 250 pounds of force**) than those who grind their teeth consciously. This is why they wake up feeling muscle ache around the jaw. This ache is due to the impact of bruxism on the jaw muscles.

- The main side effects of bruxism are TMJD and tooth wear.

- Since stress is one of the **commonest causes of bruxism**, it makes sense to reduce stressful encounters where possible. Take time off work every so often, go on holiday, and so on.

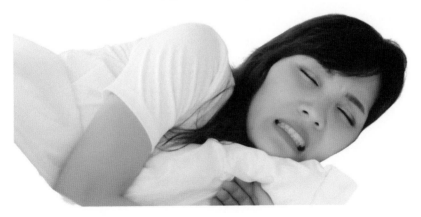

SPORTS MOUTHGUARDS

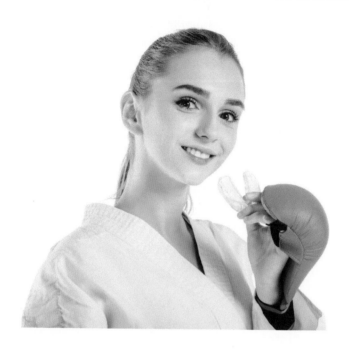

1. <u>What is a 'Sport Mouthguard?'</u>

- A **'Sport mouthguard'** is a soft plastic device used in sports to prevent oral injuries to the teeth, mouth, cheeks, tongue, and jaw.

- Over **5,000,000 teeth** are lost annually in sports-related injuries.

- When you bear that in mind, a mouthguard is essential for those partaking in collision sports such as football, hockey, boxing, etc. where risk of injury is high.

2. Types of 'Sports Mouthguards'

- There are:

    - 'Custom-made' mouthguards,

    - 'Boil and Bite mouthguards,' and

    - 'Stock mould mouthguards.'

3. Custom-Made Mouthguards

- These are individually designed in your dentist's office using a professional dental laboratory.

- Unsurprisingly, they provide the most comfortable fit and best protection.

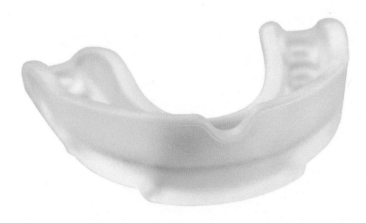

4. <u>Boil and Bite Mouthguards</u>

- These come in a pre-formed shape that can be altered by boiling the mouthguard in water, then biting into the warm plastic for a customised fit.

5. <u>Stock Mouthguards</u>

- These mouthguards are relatively cheap, and come pre-formed and ready to wear. Unfortunately, they often don't fit very well.

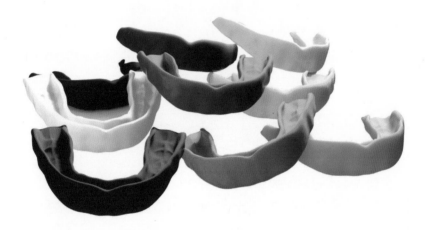

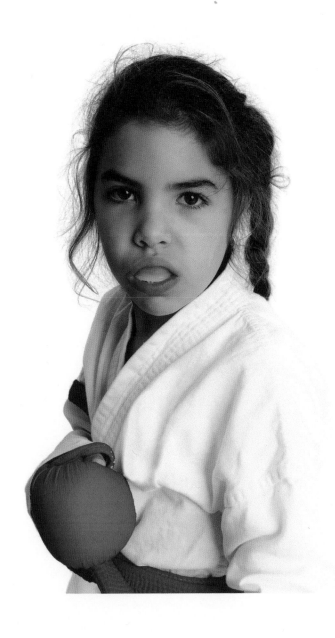

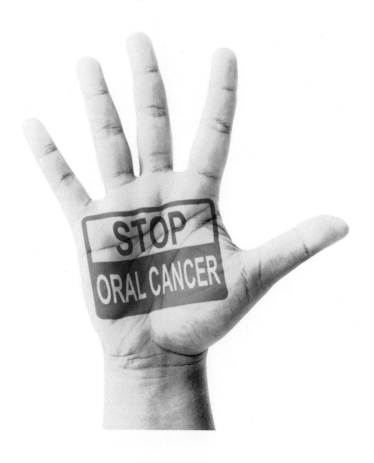

CHAPTER 6

ORAL CANCER

A FEW WORDS
ABOUT CANCER

What is A Tumour?

- Each and every one of us is made up of approximately 100,000,000,000,000 cells.

- Now for the most part, the rate at which they grow, how long these cells last, and how well they function is tightly controlled.

- In some people, however, a handful of these cells may start to grow too quickly and behave abnormally.

- This abnormality is called a 'mutation.'

- Over time, these mutated cells clump together to form an abnormal mass of tissue (or cells) that grow much quicker than they ought to. This abnormal mass of tissue is commonly referred to as a 'tumour.'

THE DEVELOPMENT OF A TUMOUR

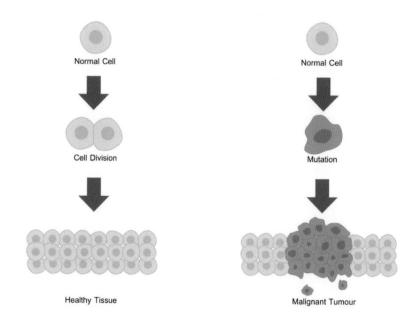

Normal Cell

Normal Cell

Cell Division

Mutation

Healthy Tissue

Malignant Tumour

ARE TUMOURS THE SAME AS CANCER?

- There are 2 types of tumours:

    - Benign (non-cancerous), and

    - Malignant (cancerous).

- The malignant ones are the ones that **cause cancer.**

- **Benign tumours** can grow in size but will not spread, and are generally **non-life threatening.** Many benign tumours are removed through surgery.

- **Malignant tumours** are potentially life-threatening. These **tumours are cancers,** in other words. They grow very rapidly and aggressively. What makes them life-threatening, however, is their ability to **spread** to other parts of the body where they can damage tissues and organs. This is why **early detection and intervention is key here.**

- Some types of **cancer do not form a tumour.** These include leukemias, most types of lymphoma, and myeloma.

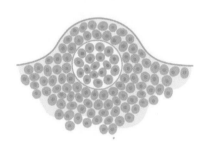

Benign tumor

- Non-cancerous
- Capsulated
- Non-invasive
- Slow growing
- Do not metastasize (spread) to other parts of the body
- Cells are normal

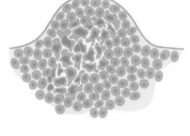

Malignant tumor

- Cancerous
- Non-capsulated
- Fast growing
- Metastasize (spread) to other parts of the body
- Cells have large, dark nuclei; may have abnormal shape

ORAL
CANCER

What is Oral Cancer?

- Oral cancer, also known as mouth cancer, is a malignant tumour which develops in any part of the mouth.

COMMON SITES FOR ORAL CANCER	LESS COMMON SITES FOR ORAL CANCER
TONGUE SURFACES	TONSILS
THE ROOF OF THE MOUTH	SALIVA GLANDS
INSIDE OF THE CHEEKS	JAW BONE
FLOOR OF THE MOUTH	HARD PALATE
LIPS	SOFT PALATE
GUMS	PHARYNX

How Common is Oral Cancer?

- Oral cancer is extremely prevalent. It's estimated that around 8500 people in UK get oral cancer each year!

What To Look Out For

Please see your <u>dentist</u> right away if some/all of the symptoms below do not improve after <u>3 weeks</u>:

- **Painful** mouth ulcers that are **not healing** or are getting worse.

- Any **white or red patches** on the lining of the mouth or tongue that **can't be scraped away**. These symptoms can indicate early signs of cancer, so they should also be checked.

- Unexplained, sudden **loose teeth or sockets** that do not heal after extractions.

- Persistent **lumps** in the mouth or the neck that do not go away.

- **Difficulty** chewing or swallowing, speaking or moving your jaw or tongue.

- A **croaky voice** or **difficulty** swallowing.

- A **sore and painful throat**.

- **Numbness, pain or tenderness** on your face, neck or in your mouth that occur without apparent cause.

- **Unintentional** weight loss.

REDUCING ORAL CANCER RISK

The exact cause of oral cancer (as with most cancers) remains unknown, but there are certainly things that can be done in order to reduce the chances of getting oral cancer:

INCREASES RISK OF ORAL CANCER	REDUCES RISK OF ORAL CANCER
SMOKING AND ALCOHOL (90% of oral cancers are due to this)	GREEN VEGETABLES (esp. Kale, Spinach, Cabbage, etc)
CHEWABLE TOBACCO (eg. Betel quid, snuff, etc)	FRUITS (esp. Apples, berries, oranges, etc)
HUMAN PAPILLOMA VIRUS (HPV) INFECTION (HPV is transmitted to the mouth and throat mostly by performing oral sex and appears to cause **about 70 percent** of oropharyngeal cancers.)	REGULAR VISITS TO THE DENTIST (Dentists and dental therapists are often the first to notice potentially cancerous growths)
AGE AND SEX (More likely if over 50 and male)	AVOID SMOKING (Avoiding tobacco also includes chewing, smokeless and snuff tobaccos, which are placed directly in the mouth)
EXCESSIVE LIGHT (Long periods of UV exposure can lead to cancer of the lip)	REDUCE EXPOSURE TO HPV (If you are already sexually active, you can protect yourself by practicing safe sex)
PREVIOUS INCIDENCE OF CANCER (People who have a history of other head and neck cancers are at greater risk of developing oral cancer).	PROTECT YOUR LIPS (If you have a history of severe sunburns, take extra care with your lips. Choose protective lip balms that contain SPF (sun protection factor).

USEFUL INFORMATION

Helpful Websites

- www.opsenuptomouthcancer.org
- www.cancerresearchuk.org
- www.cancerhelp.org.uk
- www.drinkaware.co.uk
- www.nhs.uk/conditions/mouth-cancer/
- https://www.dentalhealth.org/mouth-cancer

Helpful Phone Numbers

Cancer Research UK	0207 121 6699
Cancer Helpline	0808 800 4040
Quitline (UK)	0800 00 22 00
NHS (England)	0800 169 0 169
NHS (Wales)	0800 085 2219
NHS (Scotland)	0800 84 84 84
NHS (N Ireland)	0800 85 85 85
Asian Quitline	0800 00 22 88

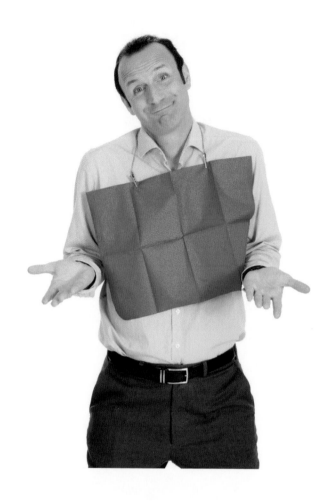

CHAPTER 7

POLITICS

DENTISTRY IN THE UNITED KINGDOM

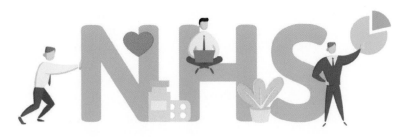

National Health Service

...It All Began in 1948....

- After World War II, this nation's dental health was worse than ever before. In fact, **over 75% of the population was wearing complete dentures back then**!!

- Something had to be done to help those who could not afford dental care (as well as medical care).

- It is for this reason why, in **1948**, the NHS was formed. When NHS healthcare started out in UK, dental care was free for all patients, but this proved financially unsustainable as time went on.

- From **1951**, many patients had to start paying for their NHS treatment albeit cheaper than the private option.

<u>...So, Where Are We Now???....</u>

- Most dental surgeries in UK these days provide **both** NHS and Private dentistry.

- The amount of NHS dentistry your local dentist provides depends on how much **funding** their practice receives from the government.

- In other words, as a general rule of thumb, the more money awarded to that practice from the government, the more NHS work they are obliged to provide.

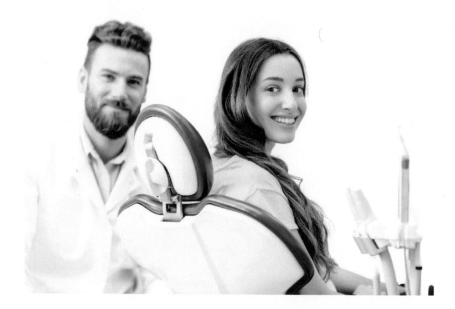

WHAT CAN YOU GET ON THE NHS?

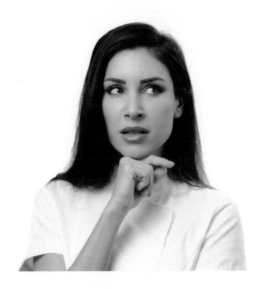

NHS Dental Charges

- At the time of writing this book, there were three NHS charge bands:

  - Band 1.

  - Band 2.

  - Band 3.

- Any treatment you receive on the NHS will fit into either 'Band 1,' Band 2, or Band 3.

- The amount of money you spend, as a paying NHS patient, will vary depending on the type of treatment you need.

Treatment Available on NHS

The table below highlights the treatments available for each band:

NHS TREATMENT	ANSWER
BAND 1	CLINICAL EXAM SCALE & POLISH RADIOGRAPHS FLUORIDE APPLICATION FISSURE SEALANT PREVENTATIVE ADVICE
BAND 2	BAND 1 PLUS: FILLINGS/RESTORATIONS ROOT CANAL WORK NON-SURGICAL GUM WORK TOOTH EXTRACTION
BAND 3	BAND 1 & 2 PLUS: CROWNS DENTURES BRIDGES

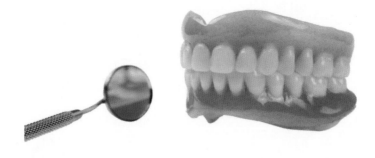

Who's Eligible for Free NHS?

The table below highlights those who are eligible for free or subsidised dental treatment on the

NHS CRITERIA	EXEMPTION
AGE	UNDER 18. 18 & FULL-TIME EDUCATION. UNDER 20 & DEPENDENT ON SOMEONE RECEIVING LOW-INCOME BENEFITS.
MEDICAL	BEING TREATED IN AN NHS HOSPITAL BY HOSPITAL DENTIST. CURRENTLY PREGNANT. HAD BABY IN LAST 12 MONTHS. MATERNITY EXEMPTION CERTIFICATE.
LOW-INCOME BENEFITS	INCOME-SUPPORT. JOBSEEKING ALLOWANCE. PENSION CREDIT. UNIVERSAL CREDIT. WORKING TAX CREDIT. INCOME-RELATED EMPLOYMENT AND SUPPORT ALLOWANCE. HOUSING BENEFIT. CHILD TAX CREDIT. NHS FAMILY TAX CREDIT HC2-CERTIFICATE.
PARTIAL EXEMPTION	PATIENTS WITH A HC3-CERTIFICATE.

WHAT ARE THE BENEFITS
OF NHS DENTISTRY??

NHS Dentistry

- The most **obvious** benefit of NHS dentistry revolves around **cost**.

- NHS treatment was designed to be **cost-effective** for the tax payer and **free** for those on the aforementioned benefits.

- There are **regulations** in place which dentists must adhere to in relation to **NHS dentistry**. These regulations were put in place to ensure optimal care for the patient.

- Examples of these regulations include:

  ➤ Providing patients with **informed consent** regarding treatment options.

  ➤ Taking adequate steps towards **optimal dental and oral hygiene for the patient.**

  ➤ Ensuring certain referral options are in place for more **specialist treatments.**

  ➤ Maintaining excellent **cross infection control** within the surgery.

IF NHS IS SO GOOD,
WHY GO PRIVATE??

Why Go Private?

- Cosmetic treatment is **not** available on the NHS. This means treatments which produce the best appearance are often not available.

- Private treatment will always provide the **best functional and cosmetic** result.

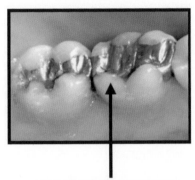

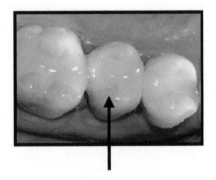

SILVER FILLINGS DONE UNDER NHS

SILVER FILLINGS REPLACED WITH WHITE ONES PRIVATELY

- Routine private appointments will often have more time allocated to them than those on the NHS. On a private basis, appointments may well be offered 'out of hours' (ie. evenings, late nights, and weekends). This means you **don't** necessarily have to take time off work to see your dentist.

The Benefits of Private Dentistry

- Unfortunately, funding within the NHS is **very limited**. Private treatments, on the other hand, give dentists complete freedom to provide the **highest standard of treatment** from both a functional as well as cosmetic standpoint.

- NHS care covers a range of basic treatments, including a scale and polish, if clinically necessary. But **'necessary'** is the key word here. If your dentist recommends a clean for more cosmetic reasons, such as **stain removal** for instance, you're likely to be asked to make an appointment with a **private hygienist.** Alternatively, the dentist would likely do this on a **private basis**.

- **Dentures, crowns, and bridges** can be done under NHS in most cases. However, when these are done privately, they are usually sent to **private laboratories** where the most experienced technicians hand make them. In addition to this, they are **noticeably more aesthetic.** Although a lot more time tends to go into making them, the work can be completed much quicker, compared to NHS lab work, due to a relatively lower demand. If a job needs to be finished quickly, therefore, it can be done privately.

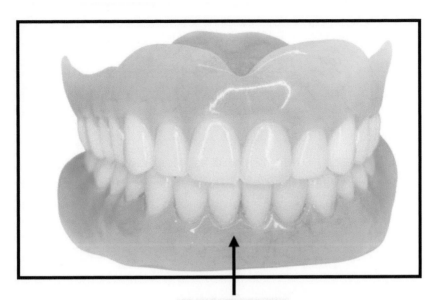

**DENTURES MADE
UNDER THE NHS**

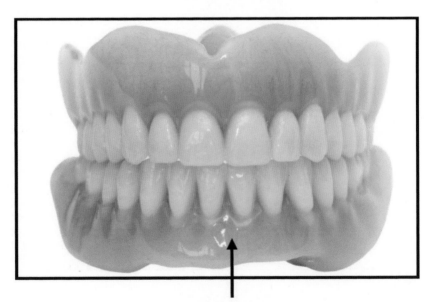

**DENTURES MADE
PRIVATELY**

Why More Dentists Are Going Private

- There are many treatments that are **not available or profitable** under the NHS such as tooth whitening, dental implants, aesthetic crowns, long-span bridges, Invisalign, snore-guards, Botox, and so on.

- You'd tend to find that appointments for private work are booked in for a **longer time period** than those for NHS appointments since there are fewer limitations financially.

- The **'freedom'** that comes with working privately takes away the pressure a lot of NHS dentists face on a daily basis. These pressures include, but are not limited to, hitting monthly targets whilst providing optimal care to patients.

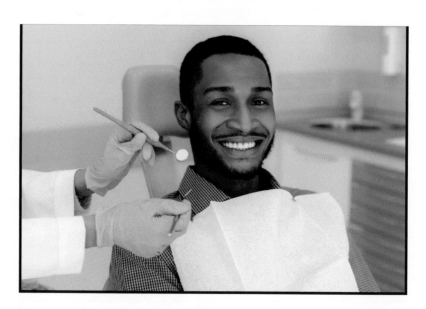

THE BOTTOM LINE

NHS vs Private

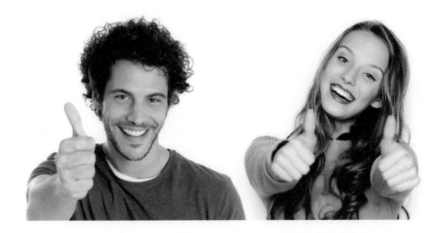

- NHS dentistry focuses on basic clinical need, prioritises oral health, and aims to eliminate dental disease and pathology.

- 'Private' dentistry shares the same overall objective as 'NHS' dentistry, but the main difference boils down to the level of service, cosmetic outcome, and the standard of treatment and materials used.

- Cosmetic treatment is only available privately. This means that the materials which produce the best appearance are often not used under the NHS.

- NHS patients can choose a private treatment option if they wish without it affecting their NHS status. Patients are often able to mix treatment options and have NHS and private work during the same course of treatment if they so wish.

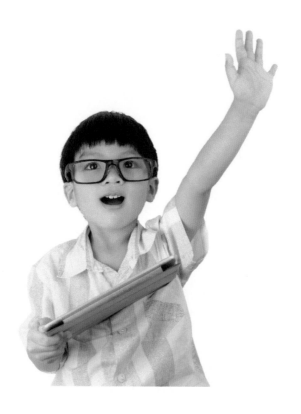

CHAPTER 8

FREQUENTLY ASKED
QUESTIONS?

Why does my dentist always stand outside the room when he takes an x-ray?

- Dental x-rays (or radiographs) help dentists detect disease or trauma that may not be visible at the surface.

- Each time a dentist uses the x-ray machine to take a radiograph, a very small amount of radiation is emitted.

- For each individual patient, the amount emitted is **extremely small**. To put this in perspective, one aeroplane flight across the country gives you more radiation exposure than the average set of routine dental X-rays.

- However, as you can no doubt imagine, a dentist taking 15 radiographs a day for 20 years, for example, would acquire a lot of radiation over time. **This is the reason why dentists leaves the room every time they take X-rays.**

I'm pregnant! If x-rays are so safe, why does my dentist refuse to take my radiographs until I've had the baby?

- Now, I'm not really supposed to say this, but it is **perfectly safe** for pregnant women to have dental x-rays. As previously mentioned, the dose of the radiation is extremely low.

- To put things into perspective, foetal exposure to more than 10 rads (unit of measurement for radiation absorption) has been linked to mental retardation and eye abnormalities. **A single X-ray exposes your baby to just 0.01 millirads.** Just to get a picture of how low that is, natural radiation from the earth and sun would expose you and your baby to around **100 millirads over the course of your entire pregnancy!**

- However, the **myth** that radiographs and x-rays cause damage to the unborn baby remains prevalent throughout dental surgeries worldwide. It is for this reason why most dentists prefer not to take routine radiographs on pregnant women unless they really have to.

I'm not in pain, why do I need a filling?

- For the most part, tooth decay elicits pain. This pain tells the patient that something's not right. Extreme sensitivity to cold, hot, or touch are common symptoms patients experience with tooth decay.

- **Some patients, however, don't go through these unpleasant experiences.** They may well remain blissfully unaware of any tooth decay whatsoever. This explains why these patients are often **shocked** when the dentist tells them they need fillings. This, again, highlights the importance of **keeping your dental check-ups regular.**

I gave up smoking last month and my gums have been bleeding ever since. Why??

- Smoking constricts the blood vessels. This constriction in itself reduces the amount of blood flowing through the gums. Unsurprisingly, therefore, the gums receive a normal amount of blood flow once you stop smoking. This often leads to some short-term bleeding of the gums as a compensatory mechanism. However, the good news is that this doesn't last.

Should I change my silver fillings to white ones to reduce risk of mercury poisoning?

- I hear this question a lot, so let's look into it. Approximately **half** of a dental amalgam filling (or silver filling) consists of liquid mercury and the other half is a powdered alloy of silver, tin, and copper. **Mercury** is used to **bind** the alloy particles together into a putty-like material (ie. **amalgam**). This later **sets,** within the tooth, into a strong, durable, and solid filling.

- A **very small** amount of mercury may be released, in the form of a vapour, inhaled, and absorbed by the lungs. Exposure to high levels of mercury vapour causes adverse effects in the brain and the kidney. However, these fillings contain very small amounts of mercury. In addition, they've been around for **over 150 years**, and there's no evidence to suggest that they pose any danger to the general population.

- However, in theory, the developing **neurological systems within foetuses and young children** are more sensitive to potential neurotoxic effects of mercury vapour from silver fillings. Although there's actually **very little clinical data** to support this, many dentists these days do **not** place amalgam fillings in pregnant women or young children.

Fluoride is bad for you! Shall I start using fluoride-free toothpaste?

- Fluoride reduces the risk of your tooth getting decayed by:

  ➤ **Remineralising** the outer enamel of the tooth making it hard again.

  ➤ Inhibiting 'enolase' enzymes to function. These enzymes are essential for decay-causing (cariogenic) bacteria to survive. This basically means fluoride helps **kill off the bugs** that cause tooth decay.

  ➤ Making the tooth surfaces **smoother** and harder for plaque to stick to it.

- People who are against fluoridation claim they have firm evidence that fluoride is harmful; but scientific analysis has not supported their claims. In saying that, however, too much fluoride can sometimes cause an unsightly condition on the tooth surfaces known as **mottled enamel.**

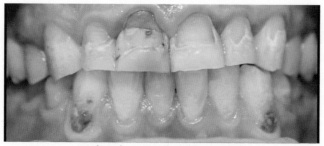

<u>Why do I get bad breath?</u>

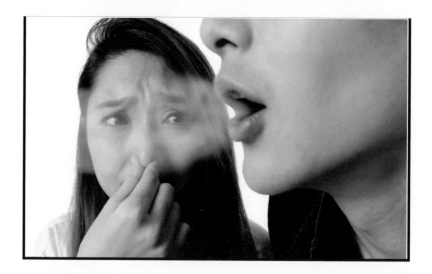

- Bad breath is usually caused by bacteria within the mouth that normally live on the surface of the tongue and in the throat.

- The 'bad breath' itself is caused by odorous **volatile sulphur compounds (VSCs)** which are released by these bacteria.

- **Regular brushing, flossing, and overall good oral hygiene measures** will reduce the amount of VSCs in your mouth.

- A mouthwash, called **'Ultradex,'** is a great adjunct for those struggling with bad breath. It actually contains ingredients which **targets and removes VSCs**.

Bad Breath vs Halitosis

- **Bad breath** is temporary and is usually caused by inadequate brushing, morning breath, or food debris left on teeth.
- **Halitosis** is a chronic condition caused by tooth decay and debris on the tongue and gums; unfortunately, halitosis cannot be resolved with simply brushing.

COMMON CAUSES OF HALITOSIS	
GUM DISEASE This is the commonest cause of halitosis. A lot of the VSC-producing bacteria are involved in causing gum disease	**DENTAL CARIES AND ABSCESS** Tooth decay and dental abscesses disproportionately increase the amount of bugs in your mouth. Bad breath results!
DRY MOUTH Saliva helps to wash your mouth, so if your body isn t making enough saliva, your breath can smell bad. Dry mouth is caused by certain medicines, alcohol, stress	**MEDICAL DISORDERS** Liver disease, kidney disease, gastroesophageal reflux disease (GERD), tonsil stones, pneumonia, diabetes, oral cancer, Sjögren s syndrome are all associated with halitosis
KETOGENIC DIETS People who decide to go on a low-carb diet or prolonged fast often produce ketones	**INFECTIONS IN THE NOSE, THROAT, OR LUNGS** It s not uncommon for respiratory conditions, such as pneumonia, to create halitosis

Does 'bleaching' damage my teeth?

- If the bleaching agent and procedure itself is carried out by a qualified professional, it should not cause any issues other than possible short-term sensitivity.

I brush my teeth all the time. Why are my gums still bleeding?

- A periodontist who lectured at Guy's Hospital when I was a student used to say, in relation to gum disease, **"the more you make them bleed in the beginning, the less they will bleed later on."** I realise how true that is now that I've had some experience seeing patients.

- You see, bleeding gums is a sign of inflammation. The inflammation, for the most part, is caused by plaque/food debris between the teeth and gums.

- Many patients, intentionally or not, avoid cleaning areas of the mouth where the gums are bleeding. Patients should instead, however, clean and brush these areas **even more** than with other regions of the mouth since **this is often where much of the plaque is situated.**

- If you're not sure however, you can get hold of **plaque-disclosing tablets** which highlight where the plaque is.

My son is 8 years old and his teeth are coming through crooked. what can I do about it?

- As mentioned in Chapter 1, adult teeth start showing themselves from the age of 6 to 13 years (with the exception of wisdom teeth). During this time, it is not uncommon for your child's teeth to look crooked and out of place.

- Orthodontic treatment (ie. braces) can fix these problems by straightening their teeth. Doing this allows your child to care for his/her teeth and gums more easily as well as improve appearance.

- If the brace is **fitted too early**, however, it can adversely affect the eruption of the adult teeth, and this can cause more problems.

- This is why the ideal age to fit braces ranges from around **12 to 14 years old**. Around this time, most of their adult teeth have come through.

- **Free** orthodontic treatment is available on the NHS for young people under the age of 18, if their dentist feels they need it.

Why are my teeth moving ?

- Our teeth are constantly moving ever so slightly and subtly from the moment they erupt. Most of the time, these movements are so slight they're barely noticeable. Day-to-day activities such as eating, talking, smiling, sneezing, and so on contribute to these movements. These factors affect the muscles of the mouth which indirectly cause these slight tooth movements.

- **More obvious and aggressive movements** may be caused by puberty (ie. **growth of the jaw with age**), and **grinding** of the teeth due to **parafunctional habits [bruxism]**. Other common causes include **gum disease, having too many teeth on a small jaw (crowding), spaces between teeth or missing teeth on the opposite jaw.** In these circumstances, it's best to seek advice from your dentist.

- Many patients complain of **tooth movement after having braces/orthodontic work done**. Once your braces are removed, and/or once you stop wearing alignment trays such as Invisalign, your teeth may start to shift back to their **old positions**. This is to be expected to some degree which is why your dentist would often make a **retainer for you to wear** at the end of the treatment. The aim of a retainer is to maintain the position of the teeth so as to prevent any unwanted tooth movement from happening.

Why are my fillings breaking and my teeth chipping?

- The real question here is two-fold:

    - Are my teeth/fillings chipping because my teeth are weak? Or

    - Are my teeth/fillings breaking because I'm biting too hard on them?

- If your **teeth are weak**, this usually means that most of the tooth has literally worn or decayed away (in which case removal of the tooth should be considered).

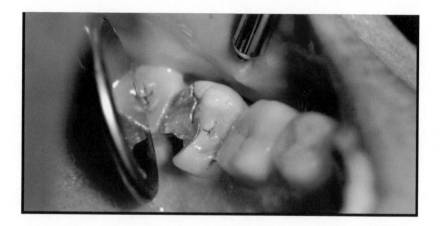

- Alternatively, if over 70% of your tooth consists of filling (especially if that tooth has been root-filled), **parts of the filling/tooth** will likely chip away at some point. Placing a crown over the tooth usually fixes this problem.

- If the problem is caused by **too much pressure or too high a biting force,** such as in the case of those patients who grind their teeth (ie. Bruxists), then a protective bite guard or splint should be considered.

My friend had dentures and she loves them. Why are mine rubbish?

- There are physiological factors that affect how well you get on with your denture(s). Examples include how much bone you have; for instance the less bone that's present, the more loose they tend to be. The material dentures are made out of plays a massive role with regards to comfort, how much saliva the patient produces affects retention, whether or not the patient has a gag reflex may inadvertently and indirectly limit retention, and the list goes on.

- However, the truth of the matter is that **dentures are not for everyone no matter how 'good' they are**. Implants, if suitable, should be considered if a patient is having consistent trouble with their dentures.

I had my tooth root-filled but had to have it pulled out the following year. Why?

- Root fillings, for a number of reasons, don't always work. There's a much higher chance of success if it's carried out by a **specialist** (ie. an endodontist).

- In addition, for the most part, a crown is needed once the root filling is complete. This is especially the case with molar teeth. Failure to provide a crown may lead to further potential damage, infection, and/or even fracture of the tooth. As a result, the tooth may, unfortunately, need to be extracted.

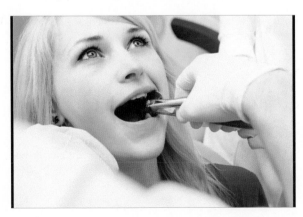

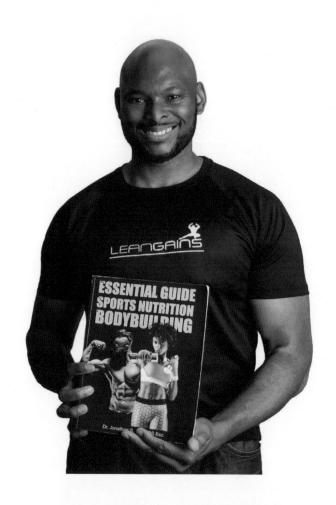

OTHER BOOKS
BY DR J S LEE?

'Lean Gains Book Collection'

Thank you so much for taking time out to read this book.

So, now you've come to the end, was I right?

Did it take an hour (or less) to get through?

As I mentioned in the beginning, in addition to my full-time career as a dental surgeon, I've also got a degree in sports nutrition as well as a background in personal training.

I've written a total of 6 health and fitness books over the years which I've entitled:

'The Lean Gains Book Collection'

Please feel free to head on over to Amazon or www.leangains.co.uk to check them out.

I wish you all the best moving forward :)

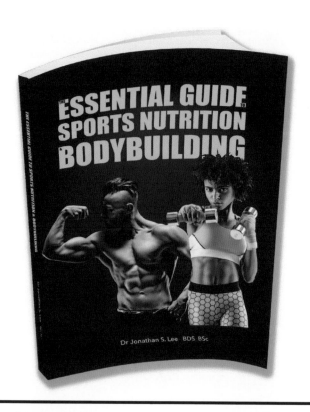

HARDBACK:	64,99 £
PAPERBACK:	49,99 £
E-BOOK:	9,99 £

(prices may vary)

AVAILABLE AT

WWW.LEANGAINS.CO.UK

and

Amazon

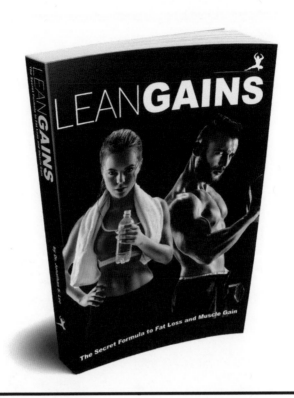

HARDBACK:	49,99 £
PAPERBACK:	45,99 £
EBOOK:	9,99 £
AUDIOBOOK	9,99 £

(prices may vary)

AVAILABLE AT

WWW.LEANGAINS.CO.UK

and

Amazon

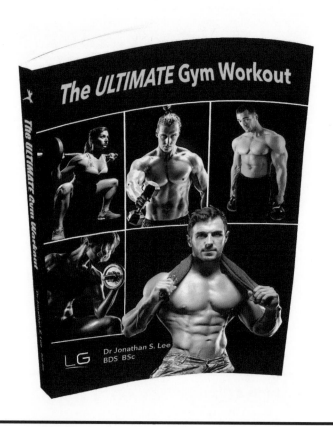

HARDBACK:	N/A
PAPERBACK:	44,99 £
EBOOK:	9,99 £

(prices may vary)

AVAILABLE AT

WWW.LEANGAINS.CO.UK

and

Amazon

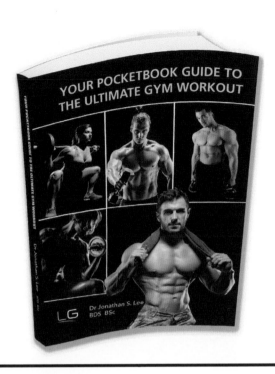

HARDBACK:	N/A
PAPERBACK:	14,99 £
EBOOK:	9,99 £

(prices may vary)

AVAILABLE AT

WWW.LEANGAINS.CO.UK

and

Amazon

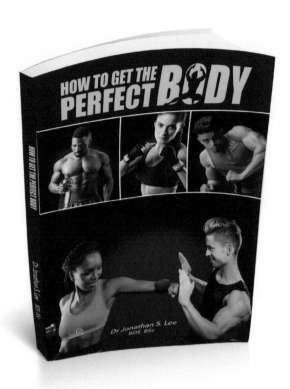

HARDBACK:	N/A
PAPERBACK:	14,99 £
EBOOK:	9,99 £

(prices may vary)

AVAILABLE AT

WWW.LEANGAINS.CO.UK

and

Amazon

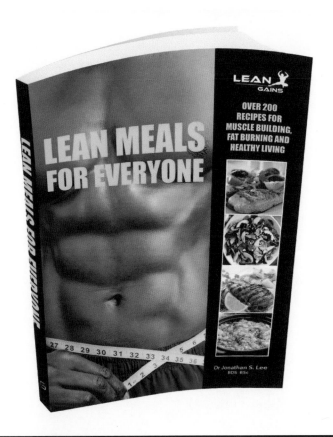

HARDBACK:	N/A
PAPERBACK:	29,99 £
EBOOK:	9,99 £

(prices may vary)

AVAILABLE AT

WWW.LEANGAINS.CO.UK

and

Amazon

REFERENCES

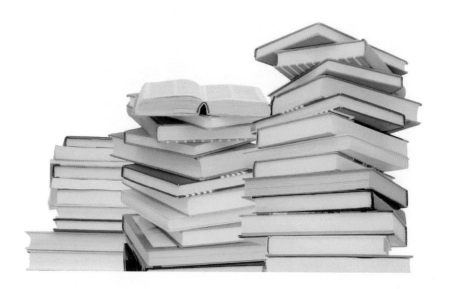

PAPERS

1.   Robert J. Genco, Wenche S. Borgnakke "Risk factors for periodontal disease"First   published: 11   April   2013 https://doi.org/10.1111/j.1600-0757.2012.00457.x

2.   DrRobert H SelwitzDDS "Dental caries" The Lancet Volume 369, Issue 9555, 6–12 January 2007, Pages 51-59

3.   Hannu Hausen, Sakari Kärkkäinen, Liisa Seppä "Application of the high-risk   strategy   to   control   dental   caries"   – https://doi.org/10.1034/j.1600-0528.2000.280104.x

4.   Domenick ThomasZeroDDS, MS "Dental Caries Process" – Dental Clinics of North America Volume 43, Issue 4, October 1999, Pages 635-664.

5.   Connie C Mobley, PhD, RD et al. "Nutrition and Dental Caries." VOLUME 47, ISSUE 2, P319-336, APRIL 01, 2003 Dental Clinics.

6.   Psoter W.J.a, c · Reid B.C.b · Katz R.V.a ."Malnutrition and Dental Caries: A   Review   of   the   Literature."   Karger   - https://doi.org/10.1159/000088178

7.   Simón-Soro Á. · Belda-Ferre P. · Cabrera-Rubio R. · Alcaraz L.D. · Mira A. . "A Tissue-Dependent Hypothesis of Dental Caries." Caries Res 2013;47:591-600. 2013, Vol.47, No. 6

8.   Whelton H. "Overview of the impact of changing global patterns of dental caries experience on caries clinical trials" in man."Journal of Dental Research   First Published July 1, 2004 al. Available at: https://journals.sagepub.com/doi/abs/10.1177/154405910408 301s06

9.   Steigenga, Jennifer T. DDS; Al-Shammari, Khalaf F. DDS, MS; Nociti, Francisco H. DDS, PhD; Misch, Carl E. DDS, MDS; Wang, Hom-Lay DDS, MSD. "Dental Implant Design and Its Relationship to Long-Term Implant Success." Implant Dentistry: December 2003 - Volume 12 - Issue 4   -   p   306-317.   Available   at:

https://journals.lww.com/implantdent/fulltext/2003/12040/dental_implant_design_and_its_relationship_to.11.aspx

10. Niklaus P. Lang, Søren Jepsen. "Implant surfaces and design " *Scientific Society Publisher Alliance*. First published: 24 July 2009. Available at:https://onlinelibrary.wiley.com/doi/abs/10.1111/j.1600-0501.2009.01771.x

11. Jemt, Torsten. "Implant Treatment in Elderly Patients" International Journal of Prosthodontics . Sep/Oct1993, Vol. 6 Issue 5, p456-461. 6p

12. A.F. Mavrogenis, R. Dimitriou, J. Parvizi, G.C. Babis "Biology of implant osseointegration" J Musculoskelet Neuronal Interact 2009; 9(2):61-71

13. "Heal Your Adrenals With Himalayan Salt." Available at:https://besynchro.com/blogs/blog/7149480-heal-your-adrenals-with-himalayan-salt

14. Ray C. Williams, D.M.D.Periodontal Disease *Med Sci Sports Exerc.* 2013   Jan;45(1):186-205.   Available at:https://www.nejm.org/doi/full/10.1056/NEJM199002083220606 February 8, 1990 N Engl J Med 1990; 322:373-382.

15. Page RC, Schroeder HE. "Pathogenesis of inflammatory periodontal disease. A summary of current work." Laboratory Investigation; a Journal of Technical Methods and Pathology, 01 Mar 1976, 34(3):235-249 PMID: 765622

1. X Xiong, P Buekens, WD Fraser, J Beck, S Offenbacher "Periodontal disease and adverse pregnancy outcomes: a systematic review." 13 January   2006   https://doi.org/10.1111/j.1471-0528.2005.00827.x

2. American Heart Association. "Added Sugars Add to Your Risk of Dying from   Heart   Disease."   Available   at: http://www.heart.org/HEARTORG/HealthyLiving/HealthyEating/Nutrition/Added-Sugars-Add-to-Your-Risk-of-Dying-from-Heart-Disease_UCM_460319_Article.jsp#.Wso6LmaZPOS

3. G. E. Rice. "Mechanisms of Tooth Eruption and Orthodontic Tooth Movements." First Published May 1, 2008 Available at: https://journals.sagepub.com/doi/abs/10.1177/154405910808 700509

4. Inger Kjær, "Mechanism of Human Tooth Eruption: Review Article Including a New Theory for Future Studies on the Eruption Process", *Scientifica*, vol. 2014, Article ID 341905, 13 pages, 2014. https://doi.org/10.1155/2014/341905

5. A. R Ness "Movement and Forces in Tooth Eruption." A Department of *Physiology, University College London, London, England. 21 October 2013.*

6. Donald B.ShumakerD.D.S., M.S. "A comparison of chronologic age and physiologic age as predictors of tooth eruption" *American Journal of Orthodontics Volume 66, Issue 1, July 1974, Pages 50-57.*

7. Van P. Thompson. "Dental ceramics and the molar crown testing ground" *J. Appl. Oral Sci. 12 (spe) 2004. Available online: https://doi.org/10.1590/S1678-77572004000500004.*

8. Smukler, Hyman; Chaibi, Mohammed "Periodontal and Dental Considerations in Clinical Crown Extension: A Rational Basis for Treatment." *International Journal of Periodontics & Restorative Dentistry . Oct1997, Vol. 17 Issue 5, p464-477. 14p.S1678-77572004000500004.*

1. JIA Li, Q Shi, Y Zeng, K Watanabe, T Taniguchi, "Pairing states of composite fermions in double-layer graphene." Nature Physics volume 15, pages 898–903 (2019)

2. C Eke, K Er, C Segebade, I Boztosun "Study of filling material of dental composites: an analytical approach using radio-activation" *Radiochimica Acta, 2018 - degruyter.com.*

3. Natalia S. Moiseeva & Anatoly A. Kunin "Clinical and laboratory evaluation of microstructural changes in the physical, mechanical and

chemical properties of dental filling materials under the influence of an electromagnetic field." *EPMA Journal volume 9, pages 47–58 (2018)*

4. G Bjørklund, B Hilt, M Dadar, U Lindh, Church EC, Klempel MC. "Neurotoxic effects of mercury exposure in dental personnel." Basic & Clinical Pharmacology & Toxicology 7 December 2018 https://doi.org/10.1111/bcpt.13199

5. F Meyer, J Enax. "A critical review of modern concepts for teeth whitening?" Dentistry journal, 2019 - mdpi.com

6. C Bersezio "Teeth whitening with 6% hydrogen peroxide and its impact on quality of life: 2 years of follow-up."Odontology Volume 107, pages 118–125 (2019)

7. Chacko Kalliath, Archana Mukunda, Meera Pynadath, Vidya Venugopal, and Jithin Prethweeraj. "Comparison between the effect of commercially available chemical teeth whitening paste and teeth whitening paste containing ingredients of herbal origin on human enamel" National Library of Medicine 2018 Apr-Jun; 39(2): 113–117. doi: 10.4103/ayu.AYU_82_18

8. R.J.Smales "Long-term survival of extensive amalgams and posterior crowns" *J of Dentistry.Volume 25, Issues 3–4, May–July 1997, Pages 225-227*

33. Marjorie L.SwartzB.S.Ralph W.PhillipsM.S. "A study of adaptation of veneers to cast gold crowns" *The Journal of Prosthetic Dentistry Volume 7, Issue 6, November 1957, Pages 817-822*

34. Je´an N.NallyD.M.D. "Experimental stress analysis of dental restorations. Part IX. Two-dimensional photoelastic stress analysis of porcelain bonded to gold crowns" *The Journal of Prosthetic Dentistry Volume 25, Issue 3, March 1971, Pages 307-316*

35. J. Wagner, "Long-term clinical performance and longevity of gold alloy vs ceramic partial crowns" *Clin Oral Invest 7, 80–85 (2003).* https://doi.org/10.1007/s00784-003-0205-8

36. West NX, Addy M, Jackson RJ, Ridge DB (1997) Dentine hypersensitivity and the placebo response. *J Clin Periodontol 24:209–215.*

37. Studer SP, Wettstein F, Lehner C, Zullo TG, Schärer P (2000) Long-term survival estimates of cast gold inlays and onlays with their analysis of failures. J Oral Rehab 27:461–472.

38. *Felden A, Schmalz G, Hiller KA (2000) "Retrospective clinical study and survival analysis on partial ceramic crowns: results up to 7 years." Clin Oral Invest 4:199–205*

39. Macaluso GM et al (1998) "Sleep bruxism is an disorder related to periodic arousals of sleep." J Dent Res 77:565

40. Lobbezoo F, Naeije M (2001) Bruxism is mainly regulated centrally and not peripherally. J Oral Rehab 25:1085–1091

41. Manfredini D, Landi N, Romagnoli M, Bosco M (2004) Psychic and occlusal factors in bruxers. Aust Dent J 49:84–89

42. Molina OF, dos Santos J Jr (2002) Hostility in TMD/bruxism patients and controls: a clinical comparison study and preliminary results. Cranio 20:282–288

43. De Laat A, Macaluso GM (2002) Sleep bruxism as a motor disorder. Mov Disord 17(suppl):S67–S69

44. Westgarth, D. How much longer does NHS dentistry have left?. *BDJ In Pract* 33, 12–15 (2020). https://doi.org/10.1038/s41404-020-0395-7

45. Boulos, M.N.K., Phillipps, G.P. Is NHS dentistry in crisis? 'Traffic light' maps of dentists distribution in England and Wales. *Int J Health Geogr* 3, 10 (2004). https://doi.org/10.1186/1476-072X-3-10

46. General Dental Council Annual Report 2002–3. [http://www.gdc-uk.org/GDC_Annual_Report.pdf]

47. Wagner MM, Robinson JM, Tsui FC, Espino JU, Hogan WR: Design of a national retail data monitor for public health surveillance. J Am Med Inform Assoc. 2003, 10 (5): 409-18. 10.1197/jamia.M1357.

48. Why there is a shortage of NHS dentists (30 July 2003). [http://news.bbc.co.uk/1/hi/health/3109915.stm]

49. What happened to NHS dentistry? (19 February 2004). [http://news.bbc.co.uk/1/hi/magazine/3502813.stm]

50. Health Professional Shortage Area – Dental Designation Criteria (US). [http://www.bhpr.hrsa.gov/shortage/hpsacritdental.htm]

51. Rutland, C. The future of private dentistry. *BDJ In Pract* 34, 20–21 (2021). https://doi.org/10.1038/s41404-021-0834-0

52. Oral Health Foundation. The State of Mouth Cancer UK Report 2020/21. Available online at: www.dentalhealth.org/thestateofmouthcancer (Accessed June 2021).

53. Walsh T, Liu J L Y, Brocklehurst P *et al*. Clinical assessment to screen for the detection of oral cavity cancer and potentially malignant disorders in apparently healthy adults (Review). *Cochrane Database of Systematic Reviews* 2013; 11: CD010173.

54. Gov.uk. Integration and innovation: working together to improve health and social care for all. Available online at: www.gov.uk/government/publications/working-together-to-improve-health-and-social-care-for-all/integration-and-innovation-working-together-to-improve-health-and-social-care-for-all-html-version (Accessed February 2021).

55. Westgarth, D. Are more associates choosing private dentistry?. *BDJ In Pract* 32, 12–16 (2019). https://doi.org/10.1038/s41404-019-0162-9

56. Rebecca Harris, Elizabeth Perkins, Robin Holt, Steve Brown, Jayne Garner, Sarah Mosedale, Phil Moss, Alan Farrier, Contracting with General Dental Services: a mixed-methods study on factors influencing

responses to contracts in English general dental practice, Health Services and Delivery Research, 10.3310/hsdr03280, 3, 28, (1-194), (2015).

57. P.S.Hull, H.V.Worthington, V.Clerehugh, R.Tsirba, R.M.Davies, J.E.Clarkson. "The reasons for tooth extractions in adults and their validation" *Eur J Clin Nutr. 2007 Dec;61 Suppl 1:S122-31.* Available at: https://doi.org/10.1016/S0300-5712(96)00029-2

58. Camila Lopes Cardoso, Moacyr Tadeu Vicente Rodrigues, Osny Ferreira Júnior, Gustavo Pompermaier Garlet, Paulo Sérgio Perri de Carvalho, Clinical Concepts of Dry Socket, Journal of Oral and Maxillofacial Surgery, Volume 68, Issue 8, 2010, Pages 1922-1932, ISSN 0278-2391, https://doi.org/10.1016/j.joms.2009.09.085. (https://www.sciencedirect.com/science/article/pii/S0278239109 018278)

BOOKS

1. Mitchell L. et al "Oxford Handbook of Clinical Dentistry."

2. Gore N.Z. and Maan R.N. "Dentistry in a Nutshell: A Practical Guide to Clinical Dentistry."

3. Smite E.D. et al "Planning and Making Crowns and Bridges."

4. Scully C. et al "Clinical Guide to Oral Diseases."

5. Davenport J.C, Basker R. et al."A Clinical Guide to Removable Partial Dentures."

6. P. Carrotte. "Clinical Guide to Endodontics."

7. Lamey P.J. et al. "A Clinical Guide to Oral Medicine."

8. Palmer R. "A Clinical Guide to Periodontology."

9. Palmer R. "Periodontology (BDJ Clinician s Guides)."

10. Sreebny L.M. "Dry Mouth, The Malevolent Symptom: A Clinical Guide."

11. Banerjee A., Watson T. "Pickard's Manual of Operative." Dentistry 9th Edition, Kindle Edition.

12. Banerjee A., Watson T. "Pickard's Guide to Minimally Invasive Operative Dentistry."

PICTURES

1. https://www.shutterstock.com/image-photo/closeup-young-woman-dentist-clinic-office-226195237

2. https://www.shutterstock.com/image-photo/broken-tooth-lower-left-molar-distolingual-58678609

3. https://www.shutterstock.com/image-photo/dentists-medical-equipment-tools-on-white-291093038

4. https://www.shutterstock.com/image-illustration/close-overview-dental-caries-prevention-isolated-302561324

5. https://www.shutterstock.com/image-illustration/molar-tooth-dental-mirror-on-white-217996333

6. https://www.shutterstock.com/image-photo/bright-picture-lovely-teenage-girl-thumbs-66547135

7. https://www.shutterstock.com/image-photo/woman-pinching-her-nose-due-bad-1761754178

8. https://www.shutterstock.com/image-photo/dental-fluorosis-termed-mottled-enamel-hypomineralization-521583421

9. https://www.shutterstock.com/image-vector/vector-isolated-illustration-malignant-benign-tumor-1483565711

10. https://www.shutterstock.com/image-vector/diagram-cancer-cell-development-normal-cells-1516206764

11. https://www.shutterstock.com/image-vector/diagram-cancer-cell-development-normal-cells-1516206764

12. https://www.shutterstock.com/image-photo/open-hand-raised-stop-oral-cancer-177881789

13. https://www.shutterstock.com/image-photo/people-gesture-style-fashion-concept-happy-402753172

14. https://www.shutterstock.com/image-photo/portrait-young-man-showing-thumbs-145076125

15. https://www.shutterstock.com/image-photo/boy-holding-tablet-raise-his-hand-657451126

16. https://www.shutterstock.com/image-photo/dentist-medical-tools-on-white-background-543467572

17. https://www.shutterstock.com/image-illustration/3d-dentist-human-teeth-toothbrush-271479668

18. https://www.shutterstock.com/image-vector/tooth-3d-render-dental-medicine-health-1935100409

19. https://www.shutterstock.com/image-illustration/dental-set-mirror-probe-tooth-concept-645120694

20. https://www.shutterstock.com/image-vector/tooth-3d-render-dental-medicine-health-1935100409

21. https://www.shutterstock.com/image-illustration/dental-set-mirror-probe-tooth-concept-645120694

22. https://www.shutterstock.com/image-photo/cropped-dentist-tools-doctor-hands-cheerful-1715643544

23. https://www.shutterstock.com/image-photo/teeth-arrangement-complete-dentures-735516676

24. https://www.shutterstock.com/image-photo/acrylic-denture-full-front-set-67374469

25. https://www.shutterstock.com/image-photo/two-acrylic-dentures-isolated-on-white-626215523

26. https://www.shutterstock.com/image-photo/artificial-teeth-on-white-background-copy-1234784620

27. https://www.shutterstock.com/image-photo/woman-thinking-hard-looking-empty-space-1894450861

28. https://www.shutterstock.com/image-photo/dentist-tools-cure-teeth-on-white-1468180043

29. https://www.shutterstock.com/image-photo/portrait-woman-toothy-smile-sitting-dental-608251247

30. https://www.shutterstock.com/image-vector/nhs-national-health-service-concept-keywords-1246573351

31. https://www.shutterstock.com/image-photo/mouth-guard-karate-1213691572

32. https://www.shutterstock.com/image-photo/patient-218929195

33. https://www.shutterstock.com/image-photo/stressed-woman-grinding-teeth-bruxism-symptoms-1081692827

34. https://www.shutterstock.com/image-photo/woman-wearing-orthodontic-silicone-trainer-invisible-1826670770

35. https://www.shutterstock.com/image-photo/teeth-whitening-woman-bleaching-dentist-clinic-1057442465

36. https://www.shutterstock.com/image-photo/collage-teeth-palette-whitening-female-isolated-1355401325

37. https://www.shutterstock.com/image-photo/girl-beautiful-smile-teeth-yellow-dirty-670781614

38. https://www.shutterstock.com/image-photo/young-cute-smiling-girl-showing-ok-121554229

39. https://www.shutterstock.com/image-photo/large-image-modern-nylon-denture-on-1375803749

40. https://www.shutterstock.com/image-photo/removable-partial-denture-close-dental-prosthetics-1859039965

41. https://www.shutterstock.com/image-photo/acrylic-dental-prosthesis-metal-retaining-elements-1666460950

42. https://www.shutterstock.com/image-illustration/3d-render-removable-partial-denture-isolated-1104023060

43. https://www.shutterstock.com/image-photo/dentures-isolate-on-white-background-acrylic-1054061981

44. https://www.shutterstock.com/image-vector/dental-jaw-dentures-false-teeth-incisors-1614252307

45. https://www.shutterstock.com/image-photo/dental-implant-retained-lower-complete-denture-1739391977

46. https://www.shutterstock.com/image-illustration/overdenture-be-seated-on-implants-ball-706523221

47. https://www.shutterstock.com/image-illustration/3d-render-jaw-teeth-dental-premolar-1043643103

48. https://www.shutterstock.com/image-illustration/dental-implant-isolated-on-white-background-1019152507

49. https://www.shutterstock.com/image-illustration/3d-render-jaw-implants-dental-bridge-1050054875

50. https://www.shutterstock.com/image-illustration/3d-render-jaw-teeth-maryland-bridge-1062905885

51. https://www.shutterstock.com/image-illustration/3d-render-jaw-dental-bridge-over-1057659086

52. https://www.shutterstock.com/image-illustration/3d-render-jaw-dental-cantilever-bridge-1535474567

53. https://www.shutterstock.com/image-illustration/dental-bridge-3-teeth-over-molar-1408362296

54. https://www.shutterstock.com/image-illustration/preparated-molar-premolar-tooth-dental-bridge-1457528492

55. https://www.shutterstock.com/image-illustration/central-incisor-preparation-process-dental-veneer-1494043001

56. https://www.shutterstock.com/image-illustration/3d-render-upper-jaw-veneers-over-1516469234

57. https://www.shutterstock.com/image-photo/before-after-full-gold-crown-capping-2099856994

58. https://www.shutterstock.com/image-photo/hollywood-smile-dental-ceramic-veneers-intraoral-1857279769

59. https://www.shutterstock.com/image-photo/outside-dental-crown-beautiful-tooth-structure-2130388616

60. https://www.shutterstock.com/image-photo/full-metal-crowns-plaster-model-1910832076

61. https://www.shutterstock.com/image-vector/root-canal-treatment-medical-vector-illustration-1435953932

62. https://www.shutterstock.com/image-vector/infographic-human-dental-crown-illustration-2144681649

63. https://www.shutterstock.com/image-illustration/white-tooth-golden-crown-on-background-133251584

64. https://www.shutterstock.com/image-photo/dental-zirkon-crown-preparation-fixation-1904990005

65. https://www.shutterstock.com/image-illustration/dental-crown-installation-process-medically-accurate-611274791

66. https://www.shutterstock.com/image-illustration/3d-render-teeth-gold-amalgam-composite-1034401807

67. https://www.shutterstock.com/image-vector/infographics-dental-caries-treatment-different-types-504131494

68. https://www.shutterstock.com/image-illustration/3d-render-teeth-gold-amalgam-composite-1035134794

69. https://www.shutterstock.com/image-photo/plaque-patient-stone-dentistry-treatment-dental-1237960759

70. https://www.shutterstock.com/image-photo/dental-caries-filling-composite-photopolymer-material-1237960810

71. https://www.shutterstock.com/image-photo/portrait-happy-young-couple-brushing-teeth-565375465

72. https://www.shutterstock.com/image-photo/portrait-happy-confident-female-dentist-245846839

73. https://www.shutterstock.com/image-photo/dentist-check-teeth-young-woman-patient-1080517373

74. https://www.shutterstock.com/image-photo/high-angle-perspective-happy-smiling-young-145685333

75. https://www.shutterstock.com/image-photo/alveolar-osteitis-dry-socket-text-list-2052302180

76. https://www.shutterstock.com/image-illustration/blood-clot-seals-off-tooth-after-1710200263

77. https://www.shutterstock.com/image-illustration/alveolits-opened-dry-soket-after-tooth-1710200236

78. https://www.shutterstock.com/image-photo/dental-splint-609111308

79. https://www.shutterstock.com/image-photo/young-woman-puts-transparent-aligner-dental-449371543

80. https://www.shutterstock.com/image-illustration/antiaging-facial-wrinkles-girl-does-exercises-1458118202

81. https://www.shutterstock.com/image-illustration/3d-rendering-tooth-antibiotic-pill-1819337927

82. https://www.shutterstock.com/image-vector/abscess-gum-diagram-illustration-1127273198

82. https://www.shutterstock.com/image-photo/young-caucasian-fitness-couple-isolated-smiles-1653543808

83. https://www.shutterstock.com/image-photo/woman-aching-jaw-holding-icepack-isolated-1858717633

84. https://www.shutterstock.com/image-illustration/oral-hygiene-scaling-root-planing-conventional-1780338605

85. https://www.shutterstock.com/image-vector/how-use-dental-floss-instruction-oral-1470509102

86. https://www.shutterstock.com/image-vector/vector-how-clean-teeth-surfaces-human-539586454

87. https://www.shutterstock.com/image-vector/how-brush-your-teeth-stepbystep-instruction-1203229621

88. https://www.shutterstock.com/image-vector/how-brush-your-teeth-vector-infographic-1145328080

89. https://www.shutterstock.com/image-photo/banner-composition-healthy-vegetarian-meal-ingredients-1716215620

90. https://www.shutterstock.com/image-photo/young-man-cigarette-isolated-on-white-401822236

91. https://www.shutterstock.com/image-photo/mouthwash-other-items-teeth-care-on-1225094131

92. https://www.shutterstock.com/image-illustration/illustration-showing-anatomy-tooth-1694225272

93. https://www.shutterstock.com/image-photo/dentist-patient-on-white-background-246463753

94. https://www.shutterstock.com/image-photo/young-african-american-man-eating-popcorns-1105128572

95. https://www.shutterstock.com/image-illustration/funny-bacteria-tooth-128574920

96. https://www.shutterstock.com/image-vector/childrens-primary-teeth-tooth-arrival-chart-2131332837

97. https://www.shutterstock.com/image-vector/permanent-adult-international-tooth-chart-vector-420714928

98. https://www.shutterstock.com/image-vector/baby-prelimanary-tooth-eruption-chart-vector-417791011

99. https://www.shutterstock.com/image-vector/teeth-types-vector-illustration-various-healthy-1749461210

100. https://www.shutterstock.com/image-vector/caries-stages-chart-development-tooth-decay-1724151628

101. https://www.shutterstock.com/image-photo/african-american-medical-doctor-woman-on-107444792

102. https://www.shutterstock.com/image-illustration/preparated-premolar-tooth-dental-crown-placement-1673668876

103. https://www.shutterstock.com/image-photo/close-smiling-woman-teeth-before-after-1455768566

104. https://www.shutterstock.com/image-photo/14-unit-zirkon-based-press-ceramic-1449582767

105. https://www.shutterstock.com/image-photo/14-unit-zirkon-based-press-ceramic-1445940392

INDEX

pulpal inflammation, 54

pulpitis, 52

    causes, 53

    irreversible, 54, 57-58, 84, 86

    reversible, 54, 55-56

remineralising, 157

retainer, 161

root apex, 59

Root Canal Treatment (RCT), 80, 85

    Procedure, 87

root fillings, 163

saliva, 28

screw-in teeth *see* implant

smoking, *77-78*, 120, 140

snacking, 27

sports mouthguards, 130

    boil and bite, 131-132

    custom-made, 131

    stock mould, 131

stain removal, 151

staining

    extrinsic, 120

    intrinsic, 121

Streptococcus Mutans (SM), 24

stress, emotional, 67

Printed in Great Britain
by Amazon

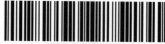

17274734R00112